# THE GODS OF LIFE

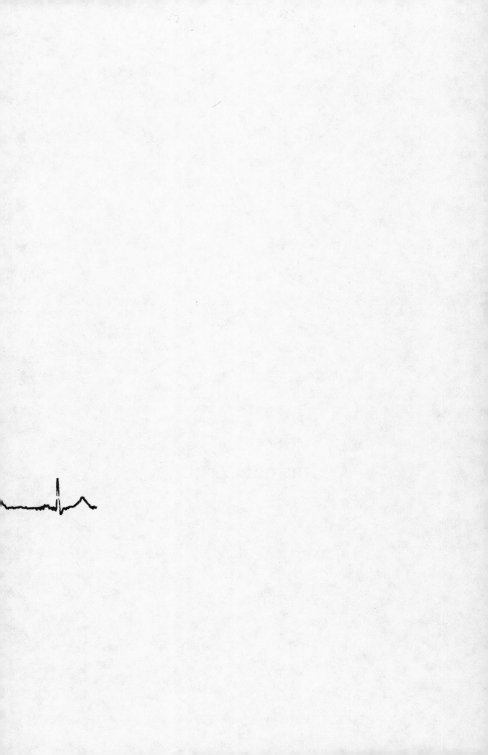

# THE GODS OF LIFE

Neil Elliott

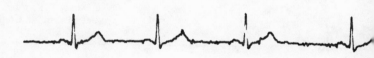

*Macmillan Publishing Co., Inc.*
NEW YORK
*Collier Macmillan Publishers*
LONDON

Macmillan Publishing Co., Inc.
866 Third Avenue
New York, N.Y. 10022
Collier-Macmillan Canada Ltd.

**Library of Congress Cataloging in Publication Data**
Elliott, Neil.
  The gods of life.

  Includes bibliographical references.
    1.  Terminal care.  2.  Euthanasia.  3.  Aged—
Medical care—United States.  4.  Aged—United States.
I.  Title.  [DNLM:  1.  Aging.  2.  Ethics, Medical.
3.  Geriatrics. WT104 E46g]
R726.8.E4        174'.24        74–11215
ISBN 0–02–535200–8

First Printing 1974

*Printed in the United States of America*

# CONTENTS

v

# CONTENTS

# Acknowledgments

Sincere thanks to attorney Luis Kutner for his unfailing guidance and assistance in all instances; to David Mackerill, matron of St. Helen's, Barnsley, England, for his expert advice and confidential insights; to Sir Alec Murray and the Lady Freda of Deepcar; to Dr. Zahava of the Rand Corporation, Washington office, and Dr. Ronald Blum of Maryland State Colleges and the University of Maryland, respectively, for their constant and interested assistance; and to all of the many other doctors, lawyers, and scientists who have given unfailingly of their time, resources, and energy. And in particular to neuro-psychiatrist Dr. William Leonard of the Chase Clinic, Village Green, Illinois, for his profound insights and learned, thoughtful suggestions and assistance in all matters.

*Everything in my life, past,*
*present, and future, is dedicated*
*to Kathleen and Victoria and*
*Stephen, my son.*

*But this book is*
*dedicated as well to*
*Sol and Helen Blum,*
*without whose basement*
*and incessant nagging*
*none of this would have*
*been possible.*

# Preface

Two patients come under the care of a doctor in a hospital. One is an old man of ninety-seven with acute pneumonia; the other a child, aged three weeks, suffering from meningocele, a condition in which membranes covering the brain and spinal cord protrude through the skull or the vertebrae.

The doctor instructs the nurse that *neither patient is to receive treatment.* Both are sure of a swift death without drugs. If the child lives, however, it will be spastic. And the old man is certainly past even the prime of his old age.

## PREFACE

Is the doctor justified in his attitude toward the child? Toward the old man? What is the nurse's obligation?

In England in 1967 it was discovered that the senior physician at a hospital in London had posted a notice for staff doctors and nurses that in cases of heart failure, the medical cards of certain categories of patients were to be labeled NTBR—Not To Be Resuscitated. These were patients over sixty-five, including those with cancer, chronic chest disease, and chronic kidney disease.

The notice had already been posted for sixteen months before the London *Times* got hold of it and made it scandalous front-page news. The ensuing publicity caused an uproar that reverberated in newspapers around the world. But generally the reaction of the English public—traditionally more tolerant of euthanasia than the American—was one of balanced sympathy. While it was generally agreed that the doctor had made a serious mistake describing in cold print the various categories of patients considered unsuitable for resuscitation, there was little inclination to regard him as a monster. Indeed, many British doctors afterward complained in professional journals that the rule which had been put in writing was fairly similar to the informal rules at many other hospitals, and they were incensed that the Ministry of Health did not defend him on these grounds.

Was this practice a monstrous one? And was the man himself a callous beast? On the contrary, there was ample testimony from former patients that the doctor was a hardworking physician, a man who took extraordinary care of his patients and who could be quite properly credited with having snatched literally thousands of elderly patients from the jaws of death.

What about other hospitals in England and the United States? Is there anything like this going on? How much do we know about it?

For as far back as we can determine in human history, it has been common practice among a great many societies to leave their old, unproductive, or helpless members out in the wilds to die of starvation or be torn apart by wild beasts, or to otherwise dispose of their aged as excess baggage. Some cultures have even developed rituals similar to the rites of spring around the execution of the aged. They have done this for a number of reasons, but primarily because community survival could be threatened by the inadequacies of the aged. The ancient Hebrews first altered this policy among the Semitic tribes of the Middle East with their veneration of the aged, which has continued, through the spread of Christianity, to influence Western thinking and attitudes to this very day.

If the aged threaten the survival of the community today, should the community "pull the tubes out"? Of course, it is claimed that in the Western world no such dire necessity exists. Or does it? It has been pointed out that the money spent on Dr. Blaiberg's transplanted heart could have saved the lives of two hundred undernourished Africans. With so many critically poor hovering at the starvation level in parts of the southern United States and Europe—within the very societies most involved in the new life-prolonging experiments —is it reasonable to spend exorbitant amounts of money on complex technological equipment that serves only to keep the patient a comatose zombie with no chance whatever of regaining permanent consciousness?

As medical technology shows no sign of reversing its progress, eventually society is going to have to come to grips with these questions. Maybe not tomorrow, perhaps not in our lifetime, but eventually. It is a part of this coming confrontation that this book hopes to explore. The treatment of the aged in former times and in more primitive societies will be examined and compared to their treatment today in modern societies. Some of the frightening new problems that have arrived with the new technology—such as the typical medical staff's strong inclination, even irresistible compulsion, to prolong dying under the misconception that they are prolonging living—will be discussed. (The progress of organ transplant and other prolongation devices has a bearing on this.) The many euthanasia controversies will be reviewed. The place of nursing homes and hospitals in caring—or, more commonly, not caring—for geriatric patients will be scrutinized. And finally the entire public health system and its entrenched doctor empire will be reconsidered together with the possibility that the new medical technology may redefine the role of doctors altogether.

Why do we age? Is rejuvenation possible? What experiments have been done along this line? Is it possible that someday the "problem" of the aged may just evaporate when the "disease" of aging is understood and destroyed? How close are we to finding a cure for aging and, consequently, to finding a true scientific immortality? A great many questions—and not many answers.

# Aging

PART I

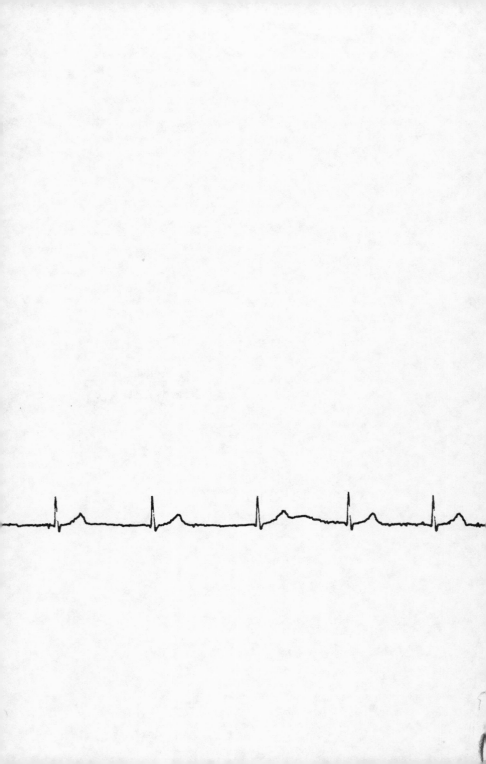

# Aging:
## What Is It?

*And what's a life?—a weary pilgrimage,*
*Whose glory in one day doth fill the stage*
*With childhood, manhood, and decrepit age.*

—Francis Quarles (1592–1644)

**THE GODS OF LIFE**

Almost everyone hates to think about aging. Doctors and social scientists are no exception. They think one shouldn't examine it too closely, as though it were the head of Medusa. "A morbid preoccupation," says one anthropologist. But the swelling ranks of the American aged and their problems have lately stimulated a number of new behavioral studies about the aging process that are more scientific than any ever done before. These studies show, among other things, that people age at very different speeds and that many changes formerly attributed to age are actually caused by other factors.

Strangely, "senile" traits are not peculiar to the aged. A group of college students and a group of the elderly were recently rated on so-called senility characteristics, and the students were found to be more neurotic, negative, dissatisfied, socially inept, and unrealistic. The students, in sum, were more senile than their elders.

In many primitive societies death was more usually associated with youth than with age, a circumstance which may seem curious. Often people did not accept death as a natural, inevitable phenomenon, but thought it occurred through blunders and oversights or was caused primarily by magic and sorcery. In primitive conditions death ordinarily struck children, youths, and persons in their prime much more frequently than the very old, for relatively small numbers lived to old age. Life more often than not was snuffed out very suddenly, rather than flickering and fading away like waning candlelight. It is little wonder, then, that under such harsh conditions the aged were considered to have some special immunity from death, for anyone who could successfully run the obstacle course that was life for many years surely had to be possessed of some fiercely powerful magic.

Today we know that all living things have a life cycle. Growth and development—unless interrupted by illness or accident—reach a peak and are followed by decline in functional ability. Aging begins when all growth stops. Theoretically, this is around eighteen to twenty years of age. Almost all functions then decline slowly. At thirty they begin deteriorating at a faster, but still modest, rate, which remains constant till death.

But the rate of aging varies considerably among individuals, and even among different parts of the body. Other considerations being equal, the life span of man appears to be genetically determined and can be predicted with reasonable accuracy using Raymond Pearl's *TIAL* index—*Total Immediate Ancestral Longevity*. This index is obtained by adding the ages of one's parents and grandparents. A marked longevity is associated with a high total—although it might be said that by the time one finds out that one has a high score, it may be quite late to enjoy the news. In any case, Pearl has shown that genetically determined factors, interacting with average environment forces, act to determine the length of a life.

We also know today that natural death in old age is determined at the moment of conception, a fact which studies of identical twins have proven. Even when twins have lived very different lives—sometimes separated for many years—there is a close resemblance in the characteristics of aging and preservation between them. If one twin has heart failure at sixty-six, the other is likely to die from the same cause within a year. If one twin has a kidney breakdown at seventy-four, the other almost certainly will have the same disorder. In this sense, predetermination has more meaning than the most scientific of us have previously allowed.

For all of us, aging is the inescapable doom, and we intuitively associate it with death. The most powerful men in the world are helpless as babes before this dread destroyer. Kings, presidents, billionaires, all must succumb. Power is nothing to age.

Despite the inevitability of death, however, the cells of the body are potentially immortal. They can be removed from the body and maintained in tissue cultures virtually indefinitely. The changes of old age are largely due to the state of balance between the tissues, in the chemistry of the body and the composition of the tissue fluids. There are also glandular changes, and there is a lower rate of living, a reduced ability to adapt to environmental changes. Particularly in the later years, the adaptability of the organs diminishes radically and they lose their ability to bounce back from stress. At the end of life the individual organs—the heart, lungs, stomach, intestines—may still be performing satisfactorily. What is lacking is reserve power. Whether or not death is caused by the aging of the heart, digestive, or connecting tissue systems, even organisms which have no such systems eventually die. Even single cells grow old and die.

It is biochemist Johan Bjorksten's idea that *almost everybody* dies essentially from aging. That is to say, we die from weakened resistance. A boy of fifteen may shrug off a cold that would be a fatal pneumonia for a man of eighty. Accordingly, it has been estimated that probably 80 percent of all deaths are at least indirectly traceable to decreased resistance as we get older. The death rate from most infections rises about 5 percent each year after the age of ten. If mortality could be retained at the ten-year-old's rate, man might have a life expectancy of eight hundred years.

As Albert Rosenfeld puts it in his excellent book, *Second Genesis:*

> Just as a man reaches a point in his chronology where his painfully accumulated store of wisdom and experience will perhaps enable him to make his major contribution to his fellow men; just at this same point where he has finished raising his children and discharged his basic social obligations, leaving him free to concentrate on whatever creative longings he has postponed; precisely at this point, his energy declines and his organism begins to deteriorate. Not only does man lose these years, but we all lose the potential products of them. No wonder George Bernard Shaw complained that youth was wasted on the young.

Though more people are living longer today, very little has been done medically to genuinely make the gradual debilitation of age any easier. In terms of senile degeneration, an old man today is still as old as an old man used to be. It is true that there is a wide range of drugs to ease pain, keep the blood flowing, and assist the sex life of the aged; there are advanced surgical techniques and anesthetics which make operations on elderly persons less risky. But no one has as yet actually found any way to slow down the process of aging.

## THE GODS OF LIFE

The average life expectancy for infants has greatly increased, but for those over the age of five the increase has been small—for those over seventy, quite negligible. In 1900, a sixty-five-year-old man could expect, on an average, to live to seventy-eight. Today this expectation has increased by only one year—to seventy-nine. And nowadays a great deal of that time may be spent in the hospital. So actually very little has been done to improve the health of the aged. Indeed, as François Bourlière, doctor of gerontology at the Paris Faculté de Médecine, points out, today a person of eighty has fewer years to live than he did in 1805—despite all the myriad wonders of modern science. Our sick cities (Bourlière calls them "termitariums") have produced an entire new degenerative pathology. Man today has softer work habits and richer eating habits. In addition, the air of our cities is scarcely fit to breathe. Such factors work relentlessly to undermine our chances for a vigorous old age.

Many different, highly speculative theories about aging are now being tested in scientific laboratories around the world. The method or methods by which the human life span will be extended depend on which, if any, of these theories turns out to be correct. Some of them have to do with genetic engineering—that is, attempts to alter the program of the cell by changing the coding on the DNA molecule. Another current favorite holds that aging occurs because certain giant molecules in human cells eventually get bound together. These immobile aggregations clog the cells, reduce their efficiency, and eventually cause them to die. Generally each investigator tends to claim that it is his field alone which will provide the true answer to the eternal riddle. It may well be, of course, that *all* of their claims are valid, and that aging is caused by many different processes. A faculty member at an American university puts it succinctly when he says:

> The people proposing aging theories remind me of the story of the seven blind men examining an elephant; to the one feeling a leg an elephant was like a tree, the one feeling the trunk thought he was like a big snake, etc.— each being correct so far as he went. So with the aging theories, each is probably correct to a certain extent.

Among the more popular theories on the causes of aging are the following:

1. Loss of irreplaceable body matter.
2. Cumulative destruction from stress.
3. Slowing down of transmission rate of impulses to brain and nervous system that eventually disorganizes the body beyond recovery.
4. Imbalance in the hormonal system; correctable through transplant or hormone addition, or stimulation of hormone-producing (endocrine) glands. (But what causes the endocrine glands themselves to age?)
5. Enzyme deterioration.
6. Antibodies attack the body's changing molecules; thus the organism commits suicide. (But what caused the molecules to age?)
7. Degeneration of connective tissue ("cross-linkage theory").
8. Gradual calcification of the entire body.

Biochemist Johan Bjorksten subscribes to the idea that we die because the nonliving parts (connective tissue) of the body tend to break down. Cartilage and the elastic fibers of the arterial walls, for example, deteriorate far in advance of the rest of the body. Such tissues are like the cement between bricks in the wall of a building.

Is there any system for retarding the aging process? Possibly, since there has as yet been no evidence that aging is basically different from other biological processes.

The genetic theory of aging holds that aging is not essentially different from other hereditary diseases, the only distinction being that while other diseases attack the susceptibilities of specific families, the "aging" disease is common to *everyone.* Families themselves show distinct differences in their susceptibility to this "disease." In some, death may be expected at age fifty-five. Others continually see their members reach eighty.

The material basis of our lives is in the sum of the biochemical processes of our cells, which are controlled by the DNA molecules. Every living thing is constructed and functions according to a detailed master plan known as the "genetic program" which is formed at the moment of conception and computerized into the DNA molecules of the nucleus of each cell. But this programming is imperfect. Therefore, according to this theory, the prevention or cure of aging lies in the correct identification of those areas of our genetic programming which tend to be faulty and break down.

According to many scientists, old age is just another disease waiting to be conquered. Comprehending such a concept may require a wrench in man's traditional outlook, but perhaps some day men will look back upon the times when we took old age for granted as "the dark ages." According to Dr. Steven Lunzer, writing in *Newsweek*:

> [Old age] is simply a disease which could be investigated, treated and prevented like any other disease. We have reached the point in scientific development where we could prevent, or at least significantly postpone, the symptoms of aging if we were willing to spend as much on aging research as on a minor war, or the exploration of another planet.

According to a famous English gerontologist, if sufficient brainpower were employed to solve the problem of aging it might be controlled like any other disease in ten or fifteen years. The doctor says:

> . . . aging appears to be a loss of information from the organism. The loss may well be cellular and could represent random attack which injects error or failure at some vital point, so that the mischief is self-aggravating. . . . If the main error is at the protein level, this has the important consequence that, while it might be very difficult to prevent escalation once error has occurred, it might just conceivably be possible to scrub the entire erroneous protein crop and return to the original specification if that is still undamaged. . . .

Aging is more universal and deadly than all other diseases combined. A great new discovery in cancer research could add only a few years to our lives, but the discovery of a cure for aging could add centuries. Few of us, of course, think of aging as a *disease*. We have been thoroughly taught that aging is "normal." This distinction between "normal" aging and "abnormal" disease inhibits research, for if aging is "normal," how can it be prevented? We feel that diseases are curable and therefore worthy of great effort. But any attempt to cure aging would seem intrinsically hopeless. One does not "cure" what is "normal." A physican explains:

> The only reason why we cannot conquer aging is that we do not try at all. We have inherited from our ancestors a desperate philosophy of nonresistance to aging . . . and now when science has finally reached the point where it *could* conquer aging, it is their spirit which rules us and prevents us from fighting for the prolongation of our youth and our life.

# In Those Good,
# Good Old Days

*They say that all this is the tale of the old men,*
*what they have dreamt in their dreams.*

—Customary ending of Iban legends, Borneo

## THE GODS OF LIFE

For most of us, old age is the age of "retirement," a time of repudiation by society. A man cannot say that he is exactly unhappy in this stage of his life, but he is certainly *in the way.* In the ages preceding our own, however, this feeling was not so common. For though his physical power was waning, an old man retained a certain exalted position in his community. As the sole master of the family's property and occupations, his was an absolute reign.

Nor was this his only source of prestige. A man garnered prestige merely from being old—for this proved that he was indeed of the fittest stock. Only a small percentage of persons in ancient societies lived (or live) to be truly "old" in the modern sense; only about 3 percent (probably a high figure) ever reached the age of sixty-five. In today's Western nations this proportion is about four times greater, roughly 10 to 13 percent. In primitive societies only 5 or 6 percent live to be over fifty. By comparison, in modern Western countries it is not uncommon for the over-fifty age group to comprise 30 percent of the population.

Scattered data do indicate, however, that even in less advanced societies a few individuals live to very considerable age. Many members of mountain societies of the Balkans, the Caucasus, and south Russia are said to have lived to well over a hundred years of age, as have American Indians and a great many other non-industrialized peoples the world over. But these are usually the exception to the general rule of an early onset of old age. Among the Bontoc Igorot of the Philippines a woman of fifty is "a mass of wrinkles from foot to forehead," and among the Bushmen of South Africa most women die at about fifty or sixty. In fact, almost every Bushman who is spoken of as being exceptionally old turns out, on investigation, to be twenty or thirty years younger than one would have supposed. Eskimos rarely live to an advanced age, the majority dying before the age of forty; a sixty-year-old Eskimo man, according to one writer, is "very decrepit."

Of course, just what is meant by the term "decrepit" may be open to varied interpretation. Most men of sixty in Western countries have some trouble with their vision, corpulence, baldness, reflexes, or mental agility. If they weren't able to wear neatly pressed clothes, eyeglasses, and false teeth, might not modern men appear equally "decrepit"? Might not the Anglo-American woman of sixty, sans brassiere or panty girdle, also appear somewhat wrinkled, loose-fleshed, sag-titted, dumpy, and, without false teeth, haglike or old-crone-ish? Primitive populations don't have our fancy gadgets to hold themselves together, and they tend to look "decrepit" somewhat earlier, but there can be little doubt that they rarely achieve considerable age. Murdock writes of the Eskimos: ". . . it is natural to suppose that the arduous and often precarious existence which they lead must prevent any great longevity."

Among animals in their native habitat old age probably never reaches the state of extreme dependence so common among human beings; with primitive man this state was—and is—also rare. Natural accidents, and the struggle to survive, tend to kill off the weak fairly swiftly, and those who do survive are generally admired as prime stock.

As people grow older and their vitality declines, they come

to rely more upon others in order to survive. Their value to society lies in their property rights and the continued performance of useful tasks—civic functions, the exercise of knowledge, the education of others, participation in politics, religion, magic, and so on. In most primitive societies the aged continue to perform useful functions until quite late in their lives. Their advice and benediction is generally sought, and the vast majority of preliterate peoples invariably turn to their elders in times of crisis. Part of the reason for this reverence lies in the role of the elder as "keeper of the flame"; in the absence of such technological marvels as the printing press and other mechanical forms of communication, the aged were—and are —the repositories and passers-on of all knowledge and rituals.

So far as we can tell, man is the only animal who communicates visions, tells stories, and relates histories. One cannot imagine an ancient opossum lecturing other opossums on the way it was in the Okefenokee Swamp back in '08. Lions may dream, for all we know, but they do not impart the visions of their dreams to other lions. Man alone communicates with complexity, philosophy, vision, detail, and imagination. He not only communicates that guns are dangerous, or that one mustn't approach crocodile-infested rivers, but he also discusses the quality and scope of existence. He is the weaver of histories par excellence. Everything is explained and given a cause in his visions—the stars were thrown into the sky by God from the embers of an ancient fire, death can come from evil demons that exist in another world, and so on. No other animal so struggles to explain his world.

Because of this trade in visions, man is also the only animal to look after his aged seriously. The ancient stories, songs, geography, history, have been guarded by them. All knowledge springs from the mouths of the old men at the campfire, and one of mankind's oldest scenes is that of the old man imparting his visions to others.

So in the simplest societies, the aged are the primary memory banks for the group, particularly for people who have no written language and no way of keeping records. The old remember where yams grow when all the rest of the desert dries up, or where to find that rather hard, unappetizing berry which is never eaten in times of plenty but which will serve in extremity. Where there are few or no written records, when everything worth knowing is carried in a man's head, a lucid mind, good memory, sound judgment, and the ability to communicate clearly carries a premium that goes beyond questions of one's physique or agility—a premium that explicitly serves the interests of the aged. Certainly in primitive societies, without significant exception, the aged are prominent as the rememberers—and consequently the *leaders*—of songs, games, dances, ceremonies, and other festivities.

Today, in the nuclear age, the situation is different. For most of us, wisdom can be found far more readily in the public libraries. Virtually everyone in Anglo-America can read and write, and few of us can fully appreciate the great value of the aged person to the preliterate community. Often the aged alone knew the ancient land boundaries, the sites of distant shrines and water holes, and the complex ritual required in the hunt. Old women were the finest technicians

THE GODS OF LIFE

in basketry and pottery, and old men were instructors in weaving and the tanning of hides. These ancient men watched the sun to keep the calendar accurate, and supervised the dates for planting, for the rites of passage, for traditional celebrations, for the rainmaking ritual, and for the harvest. They retained the knowledge of medical remedies, the setting of bones, and were sought out in supernatural matters. They interpreted dreams and advised in times of distress, and were in constant demand as instructors in anything and everything. They were the historians of the community. As Hough wrote of the Hopi Indians: "So when an old man dies there is a feeling of regret . . . for who knows whether the pictures of his brain were sufficiently impressed upon the minds of the new generation or whether they are lost forever."

Nor was the elder's knowledge respected only in mundane matters. One Hopi reported on his uncle, who had outlived three wives and was said to be over one hundred years old:

> He was nearly blind now, and somewhat deaf . . . he knew hundreds of stories out of Hopi history, and could compose almost any kind of song. Whenever he spoke we paid close attention. . . . Most of his history stories were too long. . . . But he had some first-rate stories on love-making, and the record of his life was proof of his right to speak on the subject. . . .*

The aged also have had a knack for promoting their own myths. As keepers of the community's visions, it is simple

* Walter Hough, *Hopi Indians.* Shorey, 1915.

**18**

enough for them to glorify their own roles in the tales they spin. Little wonder that in the legends of primitive societies the aged play "starring" roles. In their tales invariably the very old man or woman controlled the weather, drove away famine, invented warfare, changed stones into food, formulated the holy rites, sang the first songs, and produced fire out of the waves of the sea. It was the aged who invented dancing, discovered healing, and practiced rejuvenation. They communed with demons and gods, charmed the wild animals, and blew the caves out of sheer stone for their dwellings. Their legendary attributes were sorcery, wisdom, inventiveness, and invulnerability. In their counsel lay safety, in their service success. And woe to the knave who did not heed!

Indeed, it would seem as if the very gods had been created in the image of the aged—old people who did not share the usual infirmities of age. There is no more honorable title in the primitive community than "Old Man" or "Grandfather."

In most cultures, both primitive and modern, it would be considered a scandal if the aged were cast into the street once they were too old to be of practical use to the community. As far back as we know, the human aged have been looked after even when they were capable of doing very little.

Among our own American Indians, Lowie reported:

> The most impressive thing in the Hot Dance performance to an outsider is the extraordinary generosity with which property of all kinds is given away to the aged poor of the tribe. . . . Women can be seen staggering away under loads of blankets presented to them and their husbands.

Horses are ridden directly into the dance house and
presented to the old people.*

Among the ancient Semitic tribes it was largely the
Hebrews who undercut the traditional policy of leaving the
aged to be torn apart by the wild beasts. The Old Testament
is literally full of admonitions that the community must respect
its aged:

> The hoary head is a sign of glory . . .
> Hearken unto thy father who begat thee, and
> despise not thy mother when she is old . . .
> Thou shalt rise up before the hoary head, and
> honor the face of the old man. . . . And he that
> smiteth his father, or his mother, shall be surely
> put to death. . . .
>
> *Proverbs 16:31–32*

The aged of the Incas were supplied with food and clothing
from public storehouses, since support of the elderly was codi-
fied in the law. The Aztecs of Mexico provided for their old
people in similar fashion, and Montezuma II established what
was probably America's first "retirement village," the city of
Calhuacan, where old people were fed, clothed, and housed
at the expense of the state. Gifts to support Calhuacan came
from all parts of the empire. A great many cultures aug-
mented the diet of the aged by specifically reserving for their
use certain foods: long lists of delicious morsels were strictly

* Robert H. Lowie, *Crow Indians.* Holt, Rinehart & Winston,
1956.

**20**

forbidden to any but the old. Among the Eskimos, eggs, entrails, hearts, lungs, livers, young seals, hares, and ptarmigan grouse were reserved for the old.

The aged appear to retain their greatest prestige among herding peoples, possibly because herding requires little physical toil or mental agility, but meticulous knowledge—gained through many years of experience—of terrain. Hunting peoples are also generally respectful of the aged because of their wisdom and mystic power. According to one Eskimo: "If we did not follow their advice, we should fall ill and die." It has been reported that among the Eskimos of Point Barrow:

> Respect for the opinion of the elders is so great that the people may be said to be practically under simple elder rule. An old, feeble, tottering man, very deaf, and almost blind, was honored as "Chief." . . . Old people were always in demand for their tales, legends and general information. . . . Children spoke of their parents with the highest respect, even after death. . . .

Among the Eskimos, old men were supposed to be able to raise storms, calm a wild sea, call up or drive off birds and seals, steal men's souls, and cripple one for life. They could fly up into the heavens or dive into the bottomless deeps of the sea, remove their skins like dirty garments and put them on again (though of course anyone who saw a shaman, or medicine man, in this state would die immediately).

The Iroquois were another people who required absolute homage to the aged: "It is the will of the Great Spirit that you revere the aged, even though they be as helpless as infants. . . ." For an Iroquois son to be disrespectful of his aged mother was considered a most heinous crime. Old women had tremendous power; it was said that they could even stop a war with which they were not in sympathy. It was their boast: "We own the land." Young Omaha Indians were warned that "the youth who thinks first of himself and forgets the old will never prosper; nothing will go straight for him."

Perhaps nowhere have the aged enjoyed such great prestige as among the Palaung of Burma:

> No one dared step on the shadow of an old one lest harm befall him. The stool of a father was periodically anointed after his death, and the dutiful son often prayed to his dead father. . . . It was such a privilege and honor to be old that as soon as a girl married she was eager to appear older than her age.

In most tribes the aged were useful in the bringing up of children, and, indeed, in many cultures it has been common to give children to their grandparents. (In today's Iceland this is still a common practice, for the mother is often only a teenager herself.)

Throughout human history, the family has been the refuge for the aged. Its ties have been the firmest and most intimate, its obligations the longest-lasting. The Crow Indians had a saying, which might be equally applicable among the Navaho, the Ashanti of West Africa, or the Xosa of South Africa: "How can a man be poor when he has many children to look after him when he is old?"

Listen to this description of a typical evening scene among

the Omaha Indians where a grandfather slaps his thighs to keep time as the grandchildren dance around him: "The baby crows and jumps, and the old man sings the songs over and over again, and finally the dancers flag and sleep comes easily to the tired children. . . ." Among the Plains Indians it was common for grandparents to sing to the children in the evening, to tell them stories, and diligently educate them. Children in turn helped the aged, assisting them in otherwise difficult physical tasks, leading them about when they were blind, and looking after them even when they teased.

Many societies have tended to venerate the old, yet it is also true that among those peoples where survival was the hardest, the aged were more likely to be "put away" when their senility seriously endangered the survival of the community. In such societies the elderly had a hard time keeping up with the group, and when they became infirm it was impossible to care for them adequately. They had to accept death when they could no longer aid their children, nor their children them.

In these societies the killing of the aged was considered to be a high honor and special tribute, an honor which was eagerly anticipated and even requested by the old. (If this seems curious, consider a highly mechanized, industrial, and civilized community where even young men looked forward to death as a high "honor"—Japan in the first half of the twentieth century.)

The Eskimos treat the aged with great respect, but old people are put out of the way when their lives become burdensome to themselves and to the society. Usually this is in accordance with the wishes of the aged—and is even thought to be proof of devotion, as Margaret Mead has observed: ". . . under the circumstances of primitive Eskimo life it was ethical for a grandmother to elect to die because she was endangering the future of her children and her grandchildren, and it was not unethical for the sons and daughters to cooperate. . . ."

The Omaha Indians didn't like to abandon their aged on the prairie for fear of the vengeance of Wakanda, their god. But their ultra-feeble were customarily left at a camp site provided with shelter, sustenance, and fire. In some cases the aged were left with a growing cornfield or a supply of dried meat, with the ritual promise that the tribe would return for them in a month or so. Other Plains Indians had somewhat similar customs. Often the aged were given a choice between voluntary death or abandonment.

Nomadic peoples frequently leave the aged or senile to die in the wilds when they become too great a burden on the traveling community. A Hottentot woman, found in the desert by James Moffat, told him:

> Yes, my own children, three sons and two daughters, are gone to yonder blue mountain and have left me to die. . . . When they kill game, I am too feeble to help in carrying home the flesh. I am not able to gather wood to make a fire, and I cannot carry their children on my back as I used to.

And missionaries among the Hottentot of South Africa have reported how old people rejected their aid when they tried to rescue them:

My children have left me here to die. I am old, you see, and am no longer able to serve them. . . . It is our custom. I am nearly dead. If you saved me from this I would only have to go through the dying all over again. . . .

One missionary among the Lengua of South America presumed to rescue an old woman who was about to be killed, and received for his good intent a fierce tongue-lashing by the crone, who maintained that any attempt to prolong her life was ridiculous, and that she was ready and wanted to pass on.

Not infrequently the occasion and manner of a man's death has been regarded as more important than the death itself. Many cultures have prescribed a precise ritual killing for the aged that guarantees a successful afterlife, and in some societies the aged take the arrangements for their deaths upon themselves. The Yakut of Siberia bury their elders alive:

> . . . if a person became extremely decrepit, or if anyone became ill beyond hope of recovery, he generally begged his beloved children or relatives to bury him. Then the neighbors were called together, the best and fattest cattle were slaughtered, and a three-day feast was celebrated, during which time the one who was to die, dressed in his traveling clothes, sat in the foremost place and received from all who were present marks of respect and the best pieces of food. At the conclusion of the ceremonies the relatives chosen by him led him into a wood and suddenly thrust him into a hole previously prepared.

Some people put their aged to death in a more dramatic fashion. As recently as a thousand years ago, every Norwegian family had what was known as the "family club," specifically used for clubbing old, useless persons. Suicide was another means of ending senile life. Often an ancient warrior Indian would go on the warpath with other braves for the sole purpose of being cut down in battle. In the Chippewa tribe old men usually elected to die according to custom, with the usual dog feast and smoking of the peace pipe. At the end of the dances, songs, and chanting of prayers, a son would dispatch his father with a tomahawk "in order that he might enter the land of spirits and find himself youthful again." The Shilluk of Central Africa put their kings to death whenever they showed signs of failing health, one of which was supposed to be an incapacity to satisfy the sexual appetites of their wives. As soon as this fatal weakness manifested itself, the wives would report it.

Strangulation has been another common way of ridding communities of their more ancient members, and sometimes victims took a lively interest in the preparation and ritual for such killing. One anthropologist reported:

> An old man, whose strangulation I witnessed, was as interested as anybody in the preparations for his own death. . . . He did not seem dejected but merely remarked in English, "Me die Monday." He even set out whisky barrels and prepared the walrus thong for his execution. He was rendered insensible with drink before being dispatched.

Stabbing was another popular method. When Hooper learned of an old Chukchi woman who was stabbed by her son, and protested the terrible nature of the act, other Chukchi took him to task:

> Why should not the old woman die? Aged and feeble, weary of life, a burden to herself and others, she no longer desired to encumber the earth, and claimed of him who was her nearest kin the friendly stroke which should let out her scanty remnant of existence.*

* Lucille Hooper, *The Cahjulla Indians*. Ballena Press, 1972.

# The Aged Today

*If you knock down a child, a crowd gathers, angry and ready to lynch the driver. If you knock down an old man, the crowd blames the old man for not being faster and more aware.*

—Truck driver

*Tho' much is taken, much abides; and tho' we are not now that strength which in old days moved earth and heaven; that which we are, we are!*

—Alfred, Lord Tennyson

*Is memory impaired by age? But Themistocles knew by name all the citizens of Athens, and do you suppose that, at an advanced age, when he met Aristides he called him Lysimachus?*

—Cicero

David Sudnow reports in his excellent book *Passing On* that it is a general practice in large public hospitals to be less concerned about preserving the aged than about helping younger patients. For example, it is very rare for someone to attempt mouth-to-mouth resuscitation on anyone over forty. In large public hospitals, aged people are often declared dead after only a stethoscopic search for heartbeat. There is a noticeable lack of enthusiasm for keeping alive those who are too old or poor, or whose moral character is shadowy.

For example, one of Sudnow's cases was a woman seventy-seven years old who had been admitted to the public hospital. One doctor diagnosed leukemia, another thought it might be cancer—which diagnosis would require a more complete series of tests. According to Sudnow:

> After learning that the woman's husband visited her only once . . . and that he had been drunk at that time, it was

**29**

agreed that . . . it "didn't pay" . . . to bother with the additional tests [and] her husband's absence was stated to be a chief consideration for not rushing to make a diagnosis. His lack of concern was taken to warrant theirs, at least to the extent that she would be allowed to deteriorate further. . . . If she got worse and approached death, they agreed, there would be no point in worrying about the diagnosis. . . .

He continues:

This situation of choice, whether or not to take full efforts to treat quickly or adopt a "wait and see" attitude, is extremely common in the "care" of patients who are regarded as potential candidates for the week's tally of deceased. . . .*

In another of Sudnow's cases a small child was brought into the emergency room without a heartbeat, pulse, or respiration and was, through heroic teamwork by a large group of doctors and nurses, kept alive for eleven hours. On the same day, shortly after the arrival of the child, an old person was brought in with exactly the same symptoms. She was immediately pronounced dead. Although there was no noticeable difference in skin color or warmth of the two patients, no attempt was made to revive the old woman. In fact, the same interne who gave mouth-to-mouth resuscitation to the child pronounced the old woman dead! He told Sudnow later that

* David Sudnow, *Passing On: The Social Organization of Dying.* Prentice-Hall, 1967.

he could never bring himself to put his mouth to "an old lady like that."

There was no retirement problem before World War I, because few people survived their working lives. Between World Wars I and II there was still no significant problem, because the number of old people was still manageable within the patterns of family life. Today one of the poignant trends of American life is the gradual devaluation of older people, together with a spectacular increase in their numbers. The aged have increased from 2½ percent of the population in 1850 to 10 percent today. In England they now approach 13 percent.

What has caused the vast upsurge in the population of the aged? It may be due to a sort of "survival of the *un*fittest." Fifty years ago, as Margaret Mead points out, "the old people who were alive were active, vigorous, interesting, fascinating people—the others were dead." Indeed, the list of men who did their best work in their later years is astonishing—Jules Verne and Leonardo da Vinci are two examples. Gladstone was a political powerhouse at eighty. Goethe completed *Faust*—capturing forever the poignance of an old man resisting death—at eighty-two. Voltaire was doing his best as late as age eighty-four. Luigi Cornaro, a nobleman, showed the city of Venice how to reclaim its wasteland when he was ninety-five.

Today, however, most of the infectious diseases of the past, formerly such a dire threat to life, have been largely eliminated as a result of only two discoveries: Pasteur's discovery that most infectious disease is caused by bacteria, and the discovery of antibiotics by Florey, Fleming and Chain. Consequently, the life expectancy of young people and the middle-aged has been extended drastically—*while there has been virtually no change in life expectancy for the aged.* We might say that *more* people are living *long,* but it is not true that man is living longer. Virtually no dent has been made in the problem of aging per se. On the contrary, the life expectancy for the elderly has actually been *dropping* since 1950! While more men are living to be sixty, life expectancy after sixty has scarcely changed at all since 1789, when we first began keeping track of it. In that year a man of sixty could expect to live to be seventy-five. By 1880 he could expect to live to seventy-six. By 1950, he could expect to live to be 75.8; the figure is about the same today.

In earlier times a good proportion of those born died in infancy. The increase in infant survival has had enormous repercussions—largely evidenced in the rising numbers, *but lessened vitality,* of those who survive. Nowadays, everyone expects that old age will be debilitating. Yet in former times young people often wished to be like the vigorous, intelligent old people they knew.

As for the death rate itself, a U.S. Public Health Service report, *The Change in Mortality Trends in the United States,* shows that the death rate, previously declining since 1900, leveled off in 1953 and has not continued downward since. Now that the immunization and antibiotic revolutions have made their mark, illusionary increased longevity has been rudely halted. Despite all of the noisy trumpeting about great scientific and medical advances and the taken-for-granted claim that "men are living longer than ever before," in actual fact, life expectancy has been virtually at a standstill for some time. In fact, male life expectancy in the United States has been decreasing steadily since 1952.

Public opinion is, in general, sympathetic to the needs of the aged, but there are some signs that the fountain of compassion is beginning to run dry as larger numbers of them appear on the scene, competing in an environment which—particularly in the United States—was designed for the active and independent. The coming of the electronic age has probably done more to alter the status of the aged than any other single factor. The aged are no longer our chief storytellers. Television script writers aged twenty-five to forty probably command a disproportionate share of the public's attention—the contribution of the aged to our communications networks is virtually negligible. They write books and some magazine articles, but dominate few themes in motion picture production, virtually nothing at all in television. They are no longer our "keepers of the flame." Did anyone ever hear of them inaugurating a teenage dance? American youth has for some time been characterized by a singular lack of respect for the aged: some young people wonder if anyone over thirty has a sex life. The treatment which the aged receive from the young is crucial to their survival and well-being. Without such a sustaining symbiotic relationship, their psyches, their confidence, their general feeling of well-being, quickly disintegrate. Little wonder that insomnia is a common complaint of today's elderly.

## THE GODS OF LIFE

Interestingly enough, the aged have a lot in common with youth: they are largely unemployed, their bodies and psyches are in a process of change, and they are heavy users of drugs. When they want to marry, their families tend to disapprove. Both groups are obsessed with time. Yet the two cultures hardly ever intersect, for the young largely ignore the old and treat them with what novelist Saul Bellow calls "a kind of totalitarian cruelty, like Hitler's attitude toward the Jews." It is as though the aged were an alien race to which the young will never belong. There is often distinct discrimination against the old, which might be termed *ageism*. In its simplest form, says a Washington, D.C., psychiatrist, ageism is merely "not wanting to have all those ugly old people around." He claims that in thirty years ageism will be a problem equal to racism.

Job discrimination against the aged, and, increasingly, the middle-aged, is already a fact of American life. While nearly 40 percent of those employed are over forty-five, only 10 percent of federal retraining programs are geared to people of that age. Older people have difficulty getting bank loans, home mortgages, and automobile insurance. Often they are told falsely by auto rental companies that their renting a car is "against the law."

Treated like outsiders, the aged have increasingly clustered together for mutual support or simply for enjoyment. An increasingly popular phenomenon in the past decade is the good-sized new town that excludes persons under sixty-five. Built on cheap, outlying land, such communities offer two-bedroom homes starting at $18,000, plus refuge from urban violence, slums, and generational pressure. "I'm glad to see my children come—and gladder to see them go," is an oft-expressed sentiment in such places. According to an American doctor: "The older you get, the more you want to live with people like yourself. You want, to put it bluntly, to die with your own." But to some residents the communities are almost unnaturally homogeneous and confining: they miss their life-long friends, and the neighbors who could be relied upon in times of crisis; they discover that new friends are made less easily later in life, and that the new young people they meet do not want to know them.

The segregation of the aged has fostered a great many myths about old people that should be dispelled. People picture the aged as unproductive, impoverished, in bad health, ignored, and depressed, but the majority are stable, relatively healthy, and not nearly as lonely as people believe.

One of the commonest misconceptions is that old people are sickly. On the contrary, they average only 1.3 acute illnesses per year—about half the average for the general population. Generally the only barrier to perfect health is the aging process itself. Ill health among the aged—except during a decline toward death—is usually only a matter of diminished eyesight and hearing. One survey showed that only about 10 percent of the aged rate their health as "poor."

A study of old people in an English industrial center came up with some revealing findings: The elderly are more physically fit than is widely supposed. Over 30 percent of those over seventy have no medical difficulty whatever, and most of the remainder have only minor disabilities. The slowing of reaction time among the aged is not necessarily accompanied by a breakdown in judgment; their appraisal of situations with which they are familiar can be exceptionally shrewd. And the elderly are surprisingly adaptable to new tasks and habits. Almost 90 percent of those over sixty-five have no serious limitations on their learning ability—although many like to feign unchangeability.

Another English survey also established that health is nowhere near the first complaint of the aged. The most common complaints were:

1. Loneliness          44 percent
2. Lack of money       37 percent
3. Poor health         18 percent
4. Not enough food     11 percent

Nor are such large numbers of the aged institutionalized as is commonly supposed. Actually only 5 percent live in institutions. Nor is it true that the old are grouchy and cranky. New evidence indicates that self-satisfaction is just as high among them as it is among the young. Both are apparently more satisfied with their lives than are the harried middle-aged.

The aged are not necessarily inactive. Recent surveys indicate that people over sixty spend less time watching television than people in their twenties. Furthermore, earnings from employment are the largest source of income for those over sixty-five—not Social Security, pensions, or welfare. (Indeed, due to the great mobility between jobs, only about 10 percent of all aged employees will ever qualify for any sort of pension.) A Labor Department survey shows that older workers have attendance records up to 20 percent better than their younger co-workers—and they sustain fewer injuries.

Among the more persistent myths about our aged is that they are cut off from contact with their families. A well-known newspaper columnist probably sums up the general feeling about this myth when he says:

> The two-generation American family, usually constricted in living space, has little room for the old people, nor does it allow them any participating role. In a society of rapid change the gap in outlook between the generations is too great to leave the older people . . . their function in transmitting the mores of their culture . . . they are unprepared for the burden of leisure, and helpless when the family web has finally broken.

Simone de Beauvoir echoes this position. According to her, old age is society's "secret shame. It is even more repugnant than death itself." She says there are two categories of old people—the respected and venerable, and the dodderers, who are scorned. The French, she notes, when they go off on vacations, often "park" their old people in "rest homes," then conveniently forget to pick them up on their return, abandoning them like dogs in a kennel. She records the loneliness of those she visited in such homes: "Their eyes filled with tears when they spoke of their past lives."*

In modern Anglo-America the family unit tends increasingly to be smaller and more fragmented. The generations

* Simone De Beauvoir, *The Coming of Age: The Study of the Aging Process.* Putnam, 1972.

usually live apart, and the aged are the carriers of a dead culture. Today's small family of husband, wife, and children is in sharp contrast to the extended three-generation family which used to live together under one roof.

According to Sir George Thomson, Nobel Prize-winning physicist, people expect more privacy today, and at the same time houses are smaller and more expensive. It's harder to keep the old people at home than it once was. Parents do not want their own parents "interfering" in the management of their households, and the young do not seem enthusiastic about sharing their games, dances, and songs.

Does this mean that the aged are totally isolated from their families? Many people believe that most families find the care of the disabled aged an intolerable burden which they increasingly try to shift onto the state. "On the contrary," say those whose studies of the aged indicate that people feel a considerable fulfillment in being able to repay their parents the love and care received in childhood. Anyone who has worked in an impoverished area has seen clear evidence of this and of the determination not to part with parents even in extreme illness.

It is true, of course, that the family social milieu has taken second place to associations with others on the basis of common occupation or hobbies, or similarity of ideas and values. We are more socially mobile. Grandparents can no longer count on playing patriarch to the clan and organizing its destiny. Children may consider their advice extraneous—not welcome or unwelcome, but merely immaterial and irrelevant. They cannot be sure of being venerated, or even of being respected. The ancient dominance has dissolved in a glowing pool of future shock.

But to say that the aged are invariably out of touch with their offspring and do not benefit from contact with them is inaccurate. Sir George Thomson has been struck by the large numbers of old people in England who live with their families, a strong tradition in Britain, where in former times there was usually a "dower house" on the grounds, away from the larger house and specifically reserved for the elderly in the family.

Other surveys also disprove the prevalent concept that most old people are alienated and isolated from their families. One such survey produced the figures that 65 percent of the aged live in families, while at least 85 percent live within an hour's drive of their children. A majority of old people see their children at least once every week. Another survey produced these statistics for the percentage of children who saw their parents at least once a week:

| | |
|---|---|
| France | 81 percent |
| Sweden | 79 percent |
| West Germany | 76 percent |
| Britain | 74 percent |

Actually, about 80 percent of aged men live with relatives, usually with their wives. Sixty-seven percent of aged women live with relatives, usually their husbands or children. Less than 30 percent of the aged live alone or with nonrelatives. Many live right in the heart of a large extended family of brothers, sisters, and other close relations.

The role of the family in Western society, if no longer an

economic one, at least remains a psychological one. The family continues to provide emotional security for, even as it ignores the advice of, its elders. This is equally true for those who visit but do not live with their families. Comparison studies of the aged in England and America reveal that aged parents do indeed maintain close geographical ties with their children. They show effectively that ties of kinship play a much larger role in today's automated society than is popularly supposed. Today's social commentators persistently claim that the family has "withered away." This is most likely due to the nature of the environment which produces social commentators. As Freud assumed *ipso facto* that all men desired their mothers because *he* did, our "social commentators"—i.e., newspaper columnists and magazine editors —assume that everybody's family ties are disintegrating merely because theirs are. In fact, research shows that two-thirds of all grown children in England and America live within fifty miles of their parents; 15 percent live in the same house (and we might remember further that in this age of the telephone, distance has less meaning than it formerly did). The study indicated that Americans have *50 percent more* contact with their parents than the English. Thirty percent saw their parents daily—as against 20 percent among the English. The average in the United States was one meeting every six days. Perhaps the American sample is heavily weighted by the large immigrant population from Catholic Europe, where family ties are traditionally closer.

In sum, far from being isolated, most old people are in daily contact with relatives. About half the aged over sixty-five are married and living with spouses, and these couples are usually in close contact with relatives and friends. Another 20 percent of the aged do live alone, but usually near friends or relatives.

The European approach to dealing with the aged is characterized by extensive national pension plans which make the aged relatively independent financially, and able to live in their own homes for as long as they can. European governments also provide a great deal of public housing for the aged. Such programs are virtually nonexistent in the United States.

In Mareham-le-fen in England there is a lovely new home for the aged, practically in the center of town. Here old people have private quarters, though kitchen, lounges, and outdoor space are communal. Such housing is designed to permit the individual a measure of privacy and freedom while providing for some ease in housekeeping and safety. Apartments and cottages for the elderly are to be found all over Europe, and the aged often get special rent allowances from the government. In addition, their housing may be heavily subsidized in various ways, and thus requires only minimal rent.

Perhaps because European countries made an earlier and clearer decision to help older people to continue living independently in their own homes, Europe is far ahead of the United States in the development of community services for the aged. Generally the costs of these services—health, domestic help, recreation, food—are more economical for society than the establishment of "old-age homes." It is cheaper to help an old person care for himself at home than to care for him in a public institution.

# Decaying

## PART II

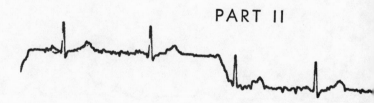

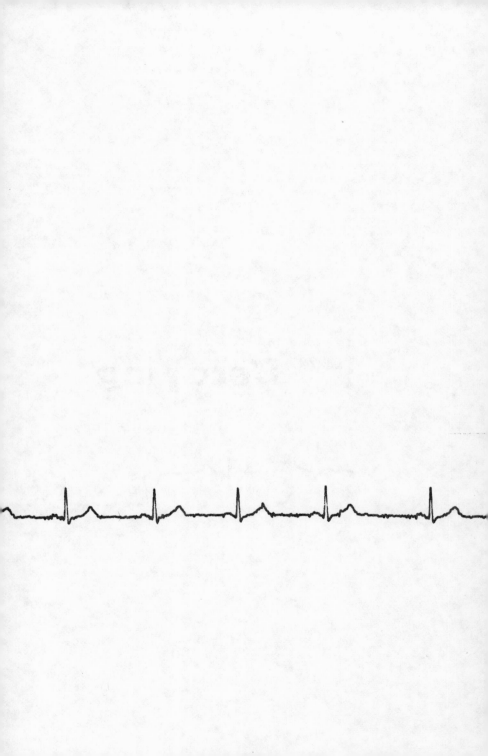

# The Specter
# in the Shadows:
## Nursing Homes

*I have seen many battles waged in court over the custody of a child, but I have searched the records of the Supreme Court in vain to find a single case where children fought for the custody of a dependent parent.*

—New York Supreme Court Justice

# THE GODS OF LIFE

*We think she's had a little heart attack.*
*But we hate to disturb the doctor on Sunday.*

—Nursing home attendant

*And wilt thou leave me thus?*
*Say nay, say nay, for shame!*

—Sir Thomas Wyatt

The problem of human obsolescence is not new, but the explosive rate of change and growth of modern technology probably has led to an earlier obsolescence than previously was the case. Who could have foreseen it—Gutenberg, in his shop? Edison, lining up his sprockets? Today we suck people dry and throw them away, like disposable beer cans. Their wisdom is not needed; it's all on microfilm anyway.

In the Dark Ages the monks cared for the sick and abandoned elderly in monasteries. During the Reformation many nonmonastic nursing homes were established. The almshouses, which developed from these homes, represented the first government involvement with the aged. Later, under the influence of the Poor Laws, British almshouses lost their religious character and took on the role of workhouse, in which poverty —considered in those enlightened days to be the result of sin—was punished with hard work. As the aged were more likely to be poor than anyone else, such workhouses contained large proportions of old people. In that respect, the workhouses were forerunners of today's nursing homes.

46

Until about 1950, people usually were sent to nursing homes only when they were sick. Accordingly, the boom in homes for the aged is a recent phenomenon. Indeed, the number of nursing homes in the United States has more than doubled since 1966. New ones are opening at the rate of about three a day. Richard M. Garvin and Robert E. Burger, in their excellent book *Where They Go to Die* (Delacorte, 1968), refer to them as "the pre-funeral homes." Many of them have impressively designed facades; some even have an imposing reception hall. Many have the advantage of large and well-laid-out grounds as well. Within, however, matters can be somewhat less attractive. A typical accommodation is almost entirely in the form of barracks-like wards and dormitories containing fifteen or more beds—some as many as fifty —set in surroundings of forbidding, cold severity. Most nursing home patients are housed in seriously dilapidated and inefficient buildings badly adapted to the needs of those they purport to serve. Very few have sprinkler systems or other adequate means of fire protection. Considering the serious drawbacks of the buildings themselves, the absence of fire protection mechanisms has often proved fatal to entire homes full of the aged, the segment of our population that has the most difficulty when trying to escape a fire.

Although nursing homes seldom have trouble finding customers, the proportion of old people who live in "homes" is not nearly as high as many people assume. According to an English sociologist, only about 5 percent of all old people in Britain are found in institutions such as psychiatric hospitals, residential homes, hospitals, and nursing homes. Yet the absolute number of this group is rising. Around 8 percent of all elderly people discharged from a hospital in England go right into nursing homes. This means a half-million new patients yearly. In the United States about one million are in "homes." Their average age is seventy-seven, and a third are over eighty-five.

How will we care for the increasing geriatric patient load? So far as anyone can tell, we won't. There isn't the manpower. Nor will the elderly be getting a fair share of the tax dollar within the foreseeable future. Although they comprise about 15 percent of the electorate, no one takes them seriously as a political force—except when they are in Congress, chairing committees.

Nursing homes today provide more beds than hospitals do; they are badly needed. But the "care" in most nursing homes is atrocious. A seventy-four-year-old woman recalls her year in a California nursing home with fear and bitterness: "It's pitiful, but nursing home people are just out for the money. That whole time I was among the living dead."

Medicare is uniform national health insurance for people over sixty-five. Its primary purpose is to pay hospital bills. (Medicaid is fifty different programs run by the fifty states to help pay the medical costs of the *poor*. Eligibility for assistance under Medicaid varies from state to state.)

Nursing homes entered the Medicare picture when Congress decided to save money. Hospitals are expensive, they reasoned, and many old people recovering from illnesses or accidents do not need such extensive service. Consequently, nursing homes and "extended care" homes were included in Medicare. Money became available for short-term stays (with a maximum of one hundred days) and posthospital care —in "extended care facilities" (ECF). Before Medicare there was no such thing as ECF, but once federal funds became available, nursing homes rushed to fill the gap, about 20 percent of them immediately qualifying as ECF. Now they can expect the federal government to pay the costs of patient care up to $40 a day. The money comes to the homes through intermediaries such as local insurance agencies.

The present reimbursement for Medicare patients is on a cost-plus basis, a formula whereby the nursing home manager is paid operating costs, plus approximately 9 percent return on his invested capital. Thus, Medicare has a tendency to promote the growth of what are in fact merely rest homes. An Oregon public health official says that calling institutions for old people nursing homes when there is no nursing service is a "hoax on the public."

In the past two decades the federal government has pursued a policy of funneling money into the nursing homes, hoping to promote superior care. This reasoning has worked as well with nursing homes as with any other subsidized industry. Nursing home operators, believing in the American system of free enterprise, have pocketed much of the subsidization and made that much more money. It has become apparent that ethical controls within the industry are not protecting either the patient or the taxpayer who foots the major share of the bill. Federal regulations have been slower to reach the nursing homes than have federal dollars. Only a few years ago, ninety nursing homes which failed to meet federal standards were paid $800,000, and they must have been the worst of the lot in order to have been noticed at all.

There is every indication, moreover, that federal money supposedly earmarked for the aged—for relief of conditions in nursing homes—is often sidetracked to state treasuries or to the very many physicians who own nursing homes—while simultaneously earning more than $30,000 yearly from Medicare. In many states these same doctors are sitting on the local boards that are supposed to regulate nursing homes. A recent Senate investigation revealed that the head of Medicare in one state was also the director of a chain of nursing homes.

Recently, the Social Security Administration took action against twenty nursing homes in Florida, New York, Arizona, and Illinois that had cheated the government out of $4 million in Medicare money. Several had billed fraudulently, others had billed for services that had not been medically necessary. When such cases are uncovered, the nursing homes are sometimes given the opportunity to repay in kind—to make up the overcharge—by offering free services to future patients. More frequently, repayment from the homes is "negotiated" —HEW accepts forty cents on the dollar in greatly inflated charges for future Medicare patients. Crooked nursing home administrators can thus get away clean. They chance little if they get caught, and the profits can be considerable. One nursing home operator owing $500,000 to Medicare merely closed his doors and started another home elsewhere!

Physicians have been investing heavily in nursing homes. A precise account of how many are involved is difficult to compile because many doctors register their holdings in the names of friends and relatives, certainly a curious practice for "professional" men. As doctors are most often the people who recommend nursing homes, there has been some question of conflict of interest.

How is it that such chicanery is allowed to get by? Why doesn't someone file a criminal suit for fraud? Unfortunately, responsibility for nursing homes is divided among several different agencies, and inspection is the responsibility of the fifty separate states; there is virtually no federal control, and bribery is said to be widespread.

Then how does Washington verify the operating costs and the "invested capital" as claimed by the nursing homes? It doesn't. Rarely has a setup been more promising for impropriety. Medicare is responsible for spending around $500 million of our money yearly, with virtually no accounting procedure worthy of note. What the Medicare intermediaries do is to watch for unusual amounts of physical therapy, abnormally large numbers of bills for physician visits, and more patient treatments than a doctor would normally be likely to perform. One physician, for example, submitted bills for patients who had long been dead. Another charged full fees for seeing twenty patients in twenty minutes.

The possibilities for profit are intriguing. Lest anyone suppose that nursing homes are not profit-making ventures, we need only note that some *seventy* chain operations are selling stock on Wall Street. In England most nursing homes are nonprofit. In the United States the situation is reversed; around 90 percent are business ventures. Mutual fund companies have so much faith in the profitability of nursing homes that they own over six million shares of stock in nursing home chains. These stocks were once known as "the hottest on Wall Street." At least a part of the attraction is the belief that the elderly will be an increased percentage of our population in coming years. Although this theory has been statistically off base since 1950, it does seem as if nursing homes will be a "final solution" for increasing numbers of the aged.

The vast majority of entrepreneurs going into the nursing home "business" are not distinguishable from other businessmen. Previously, they may have been builders, contractors, or restaurant owners. Few of the nursing home chains that have "gone public" are headed by health care experts. Medicenters, Inc., was financed by the developers of Holiday Inns, the motel chain. Another outfit is the Four Seasons chain, which operates more than fifty nursing homes across the United States, at an estimated profit of $1,000 per bed per year before taxes—and no wonder, with the cost of a decent nursing home running upwards of $700 per month.

Arkansas Congressman David Pryor recently visited twelve nursing homes near Washington, D.C. "I found only two where I would be willing to send my mother," he reported later to Congress, "but I don't think I could afford either one of those on my forty-two thousand, five hundred dollar salary."

The nursing home public gets very little for its money. Seventy-five percent of all patients do not see a doctor for six months. The average amount of doctor care per patient amounts to only two and one-half minutes per week. *Only about half of the homes have any nurses on duty,* a situation a Los Angeles administrator explains as an economy move.

*Drugs in nursing homes are usually administered improperly* and are commonly used to "docile" patients. They are administered by almost anybody, including the cleaning woman. More Medicare money is spent on tranquilizers than any other sort of medicine, a fact that seems particularly interesting when we note the American Nursing Home Association's assertion that 50 percent of all patients are "confused" all or part of the time.

*Nursing homes are firetraps;* in a recent estimate, thousands of homes did not meet minimum health and fire safety standards. The National Fire Prevention Association claims that nursing homes are the most dangerous places in the nation in which to live. Fires are disastrous, for inmates are the least mobile portion of our population. Not long ago, thirty-two persons died in a home in Marietta, Ohio, that was supposed to be "one of the best." *Reported* nursing home fires occur more than once every day. Most states do not require sprinkler systems, which is the only real protection for the bedridden. Fire reports frequently note "no attendant on duty." Few homes have adequate fire drills or adequately regulate smoking in bed (fully half of all fires are caused by cigarettes lit by patients prone to falling asleep while smoking).

*Nursing home administrators need have no specific qualifications,* and, indeed, even "nurses" with very irregular qualifications are hired. In *all* states, nurses may be approved via "waiver"—which often means that a "very nice lady" is "head nurse" even when she has had no nurse's training whatever.

To top it all, *the food served to the average patient costs less than one dollar per day.*

The Social Security Administration—which administers Medicare—must approve nursing homes, but here too the Medicare standards, which in many respects are vague and subject to a wide range of interpretations, are actually applied by state and county agencies. These agencies' reports on the homes are sent to the regional office of the Social Security Administration where certifications are signed with little or no knowledge of actual conditions. Not that the Medicare administrators don't know how many facilities are deficient under their standards—they do. The proportion is about 75 percent of all homes.

Unfortunately, welfare funds to substandard homes have rarely been cut off by state agencies. The usual subterfuge is to allow a "grace" period for compliance. A December, 1966, study by the federal General Accounting Office revealed that ". . . steps to revoke licenses had not been taken even after inordinately long prevalence of violations of state law . . . numerous cases of overcrowding, inadequate nursing supervision, incomplete patient records, illegal administration of drugs, and unclean and poorly maintained facilities. . . ." A hospital administrator in Tennessee states: "If the State of Tennessee would be as firm as it could be, I would wager that 50 percent of the nursing homes would be closed down overnight. But then where would these people [the patients] go?" A Florida official states categorically: "We've never had the appropriations necessary to enforce the law." In Florida there are several hundred nursing homes—but only two inspectors in the entire state. In Wisconsin one 317-bed home went without regular state inspections for more than three years—then a routine check turned up a list of violations four pages long.

"Bad" nursing homes can be really inhuman. Patients are often locked in their rooms or tied to chairs. Again, less than one dollar per day is spent on their food. Drugs are used without prescription and indiscriminately. Addicts are attracted to work in such places in order to gain access to a pharmacy. A typical letter of complaint to a Congressman reads:

I saw attendants ignore one old woman's call for help; I saw one owner talk in an insultingly derogatory way about a patient, in front of that very patient; I saw incredible filth and signs of neglect; and I heard things that seemed to me to evidence a callousness and crudity that I certainly wouldn't want any parents of mine exposed to. The owner of the home said to me, "Look, your father is getting old and he is hard to handle, right? You bring him in here, maybe in a few weeks you can take him home on a Sunday afternoon, but the first thing is you've got to show these old people you're the boss."

The nursing home industry has been quick to foist on the public the impression that nursing homes are strictly licensed, duly inspected, and that at all times a health team is physically present or at least near enough to serve. Not true. Licensing is a negligible factor in regulating nursing homes, since most licensing agencies can't be bothered to put the homes through any sort of examination. If the fee is paid, the home gets a license. Thus the licensing board is strictly a revenue producer for the state. In some states it is as easy to open a nursing home as it is to open a gas station; in some, even easier. Inspection after operation commences is a joke. *Most* states make no allowance whatever for inspection. Among those which do, inspection is chaotic, vastly under-manned, and subject to bribery.

Only 10 percent of all nursing home administrators have any training whatever for their jobs. Only a third have a college degree. Lower-echelon staff, particularly the nurses' aides and orderlies, are rarely paid above the minimum federal wage. Most of them have less training and experience for their jobs than the average restaurant dishwasher, and their turnover is as great, if not greater. Since the nurses' aides and orderlies have the closest contact with the patient—indeed, they are the most frequent dispensers of medicine—it would seem dangerous that so few of them have had any training other than "on the job."

The California Association of Nursing Homes emphasizes that *those homes on its membership list* pay wages of $20 million yearly. This would seem impressive, except for the fact that, with 7,500 employees, this comes to a per capita income of only $2,650—in California, with one of the United States' highest wage and cost-of-living structures.

It's true, of course, that both the Medicare and Medicaid agencies of HEW issue standards for nursing homes participating in their programs. However, neither agency applies their standards or does any inspecting. In the case of Medicaid, which is a state-administered program, nursing homes are certified for participation in the program by state agencies. Often the approval of these agencies is based on the surveys and reports made by county agencies. But the federal administrative agency, the Social and Rehabilitative Service, has virtually no control over the quality or frequency of these surveys and does not even receive information on the number of homes certified by the states. In a hearing before the Intergovernmental Relations Senate Subcommittee on Government Operations it was recently disclosed that Social Security officials have *no* information on the qualifications of surveyors doing Medicare inspections! They don't even know to what extent the inspections are done by state personnel or county personnel!

As a practical matter, then, the federal government has no way at all of knowing whether its standards are being met. If a patient or his family writes to his representative in Congress to complain of conditions in a Medicaid nursing home, the complaint is referred to HEW for investigation. But from there it is merely referred to the state agency and from there to the county agency—which is probably responsible for permitting the violations in the first place!

The patient has nowhere to turn, for no one is really in control. What little jurisdiction exists is highly fragmented. Considering the fact that two-thirds of all patients are maintained in the homes by federal money, this is a remarkable state of affairs. The cost to the American taxpayer is approximately $2 billion each year, and there is virtually no control over where this money is going.

Unlike Medicare, Medicaid does provide for long-term care. Medicaid programs in most states pay about $12 a day for care. What this means is that the poor can now receive care in the cheapest homes, the wealthy can afford the best—but the middle class can afford nothing. They can neither pay the $30 per day for a good home, nor can they qualify for public assistance. Their only solution is to liquidate their assets by paying their own way in nursing homes for as long as they can afford it. Once their assets are gone, they go "on welfare." Then the American system "helps" them.

But the aged person's problems are not solved even if he is able to afford the basic charges of a nursing home. They may be just beginning. Most nursing homes, when discussing prices, are prone to state a flat monthly charge while conveniently forgetting the vast number of "additionals" that will be imposed once the patient is in their clutches. The average, unknowledgeable person assumes that the monthly fee will include most ordinary requirements of old people. Few nursing homes show their price list of "options" until after the patient has been lured into moving in. The first bill contains shocking surprises. Starting with a basic charge of $600 a month for a single room with meals, incredible and overpriced extras may be added such as:

| | |
|---|---|
| Admission sets | $ 3.50 |
| Air mattress | $45.00/month |
| Air worms | $ 3.50 |
| Oxygen | $30.00/tank |
| Television | $21.00/month |

Paying extra for "admission sets" amounts to the patient paying separately for the home's routine office work. Certainly the charge for "air mattress" is a ridiculously inflated one.

The price for oxygen is about double the standard. And as television sets can be bought most anywhere for $100, the rental exacted is patent gouging of the helpless patient. As for "air worms" expense, that was undoubtedly made up. Furthermore, we should question the basic rental itself. Is $600 for room and board, without any other extras, a reasonable rent anywhere in the United States? Incidentally, charges for services not really rendered are commonplace. And patients have even been confined to their beds because "bed care" entitles the nursing home owners to $3 or $4 more per day.

But the most ruthless method of gouging indulged in by the nursing homes is not the padded bill; it is the life-care contract. This, as found in American nursing homes, is totally unlike anything found in nursing homes anywhere else in Western civilization. Briefly, the usual "life" contract obliges the individual joining a nursing home to sign over his entire estate to the proprietors in return for guaranteed care for the rest of his life. As Garvin and Burger put it in *Where They Go to Die*:

> . . . the home is in the unusual position of being able to control the terms of the contract. How much care is "care"? How much should be spent on rehabilitation, if anything? When should a doctor be called in? In practice, simple day-to-day decisions are obviously influenced by the fact that *everything the home pays out for the benefit of the patient works against the profits of the home.* [italics theirs]

There has been some discussion as to whether or not the life-care patient is not hastening his own demise by putting a nursing home in a position where it will profit from his death. It is not so difficult for a nurse ministering to a life-care patient to move to the telephone just a little more slowly. Or to forget to administer medicine. Or to serve a slightly smaller tray of food. No one would call it murder.

Say Garvin and Burger:

> It is not overstating it to say that some nursing homes find it expedient to hasten the death of their patients. This need not happen suddenly. It may even seem to be merciful . . . the typical patient is over eighty, bedridden, in pain for the greater part of the day, and scarcely aware of what is happening around him. Add to this situation the fact that the nursing home may be desperately in need of the funds of the patient or, if these have already been turned over . . . the bed space. Everything points to the desirability of abbreviating the life of the patient. . . . Many homes, consciously or unconsciously, have a chilling policy of "not letting older patients linger on." In the case of life-care patients, the policy is likely to be a conscious one . . . the very nature of the life contract is that the home benefits when it does the very opposite of what you require of a nursing home: namely, when it accepts patients with the expectation of an early death.

They explain how the homes gradually break the life-care patient's spirit. He may be confined to his room for being noisy, spanked like a child, kept from his favorite pastimes, threatened, and teased. He may be ostracized by turning other patients against him. Mail can be carefully delayed or forgotten. Attendants may be unduly rough and critical, annoyed at the patient's helpless incontinence, whispering in his ear that his family is no longer interested in visiting. "Heartsickness" can kill an aged patient faster than any known malady. According to Dr. W. N. Leak, writing in *The Practitioner*:

> . . . the real secret of treating any old people is to let them have their own way, or to make them think they are getting it. There is no surer way of rapidly finishing off an old patient than to impose on him a strict regime of any kind, whether dietary, medicinal or even just insisting on his bed being kept immaculate. In such circumstances old people . . . slide away in spite of all medical and nursing care. Relax the reins . . . and it is extraordinary how often they will pick up. . . .

It has been said that the nursing home industry today parallels to some degree the early days of hospital development in the United States, when hospitals were also business companies. Hospital regulation eventually served to change this direction toward locally sponsored nonprofit hospital groups. Is this the future, too, for nursing homes?

# The Other Specter:
## Hospitals

*They all died during the day today, lucky us, so you'll probably have it nice and easy.*

—Day nurse to night nurse

DECAYING

*What do you know about him? He wept the other day after you walked away, fat tears of frustration because you talked to him like a child and his paralytic tongue couldn't answer.*

—Patient's son to nurse

Most Americans, nearly 75 percent, are routinely processed "out" of life through the labyrinthine and antiseptic corridors of the hospitals. The situation is quite the reverse in England, where the majority prefer to die at home, among their loved ones, but the percentage is decreasing. The number of terminal patients in hospital care is escalating wildly, cancer patients being the largest single group among them (about 80 percent of the total terminal care population). In addition, there are large numbers of patients with severe chest disease, cerebral stroke, or some other acute or subacute disease which fails to respond to treatment. In England, as well as in America, the geriatrics beds in hospitals are always full, and there is a lengthy waiting list. The unavailability of long-stay beds can be expected to increase, and many acute beds will eventually be taken up by the long-stays, or "chronics."

If old people in former times seemed more vigorous and healthy than they are today, it was because they actually were—only the strongest survived to a ripe old age. Today, however, with the traditional diseases of youth and middle age all but conquered, a very large proportion of our population is living long enough to become susceptible to that class of diseases known as *chronic*. Cancer, heart disease, stroke, paralysis, are slow diseases which take a long time to kill,

63

diseases which lead to chronic invalidism. Consequently our hospitals today are full of starved-looking creatures asleep or half-awake on some narcotic. Some mumble, others complain of pain. Some are too feeble to raise a cup of water to their dying lips. Paralytics in filthy diapers cry to nurses for help and are scolded for being "dirty." The vast majority of these chronics will never leave the hospital, but will deteriorate still further as a result of the treatment they receive. According to a nursing officer in the Scottish Home and Health Department: ". . . as much as one-third of the patients who are admitted as a matter of expediency are made into nursing cases by the environment." A doctor points out:

> In 70 percent of cases, nocturnal confusion and restlessness in old people is caused by physical rather than mental troubles. But a busy houseman in a general ward may pass this symptom off as senility and mental decay where more often the reason is constipation. He is then apt to prescribe a barbiturate sedative which, if given in normal adult doses to old people, often increases confusion and leads to depression and incontinence.

Some of these "chronic" cases should never have been hospitalized in the first place. A New York City physician who has studied cancer diagnoses states:

> The mass crowding of a group of patients labeled "terminal" . . . constitutes a grave danger . . . it seems reasonable to conclude that a fresh evaluation of . . . mental institutions, institutions for chronic care, or homes for the incurably sick, would unearth a rewarding number

of salvageable patients who can be returned to their normal place in society . . . we were especially interested in those with a diagnosis of advanced cancer. In a number of these patients, major errors in diagnosis or management were encountered.

And cancer is an illness in which errors in diagnosis are ordinarily minimal.


Although the United States is at the top of the world economically, statistics show it to be very far down the list of advanced nations in virtually all measurable aspects of public health. In fact, the health of most Americans is worse today than it was fifteen or twenty years ago, according to the Committee for National Health Insurance. Deaths of women in childbirth have increased sharply since 1952; we are fourteenth in infant mortality and eighteenth in life expectancy for males. Despite all propaganda to the contrary in the public press, life expectancy is falling in all categories, particularly for males.

Thus, although we spend more money per capita than any other country on doctors' fees and other medical expenses (roughly 8 percent of our GNP), we rank only seventeenth in the world in the quality of health care. Britain, which spends only 4 percent of her Gross National Product on health, ranks much higher. We can credit our inferior situation to our haphazard, cut-and-paste, laissez-faire medical system. One of the major culprits is the hospital.

Isn't one at least assured of superior care at the more

expensive hospitals? No. The English survey *Patients and Their Hospitals* found no correlation whatever between contentment of the patient and hospital cost. Indeed, the hospital with the most contented patients had by far the lowest charges.

The senile elderly are often not admitted to good nursing homes because they are sick, require a good deal of attention, and are less likely than any other group to be able to pay. Often they end up in state mental hospitals, "bad" nursing homes, or in the geriatric wings of public hospitals.

In both England and America approximately 40 percent of those interred in mental hospitals are not "mentally ill" at all, but merely aged and senile. In Barbara Robb's definitive work, *Sans Everything*, Dr. Stephen Horsley states: "Perhaps 80 percent of elderly patients in mental hospitals have mental symptoms attributable to untreated *physical* ailments." A *Time* magazine article somewhat corroborates this by reminding us that: ". . . studies have shown that the percentage of psychiatric impairment of old persons is no greater than that for younger groups. But younger people are usually treated if their psychological problems are severe."

According to a New York psychologist, when we find unusual nervousness, irritability, or depression in a young person, or unaccountable anger, apathy, or personality change, we make sure that he sees a physician. But in elderly people these symptoms are considered par for the course. We often fail to consider the possibility that elderly people can recover. (We might note in passing that the rate of mental disorders actually *declines* after seventy.) The prospect of being sent to a geriatric ward is not very cheering either. About 30 percent of all such patients die within three months. Several years ago, the English magazine *Nursing Mirror* reported on a meeting of the English Royal College of Nursing and the American Nurses' Association at which it was agreed that if nurses were sent for geriatrics training to any but a very few hospitals or geriatric wards they would pick up only bad habits. Listen to this letter to the *Nursing Mirror* in which nurse Pearl L. Foster describes the state of an elderly woman patient in a hospital after a stroke:

> She was in a low chair very nearly falling off the seat; her paralyzed arm was hanging over the side; a blanket had been thrown over her shoulders, but she had no covering at all from the pelvis downwards. The patient said she had been like this for three hours and longed to be back in bed. . . . I asked that she be returned to her bed. . . . When we [returned] I was shattered to see how the patient had been left. . . . I found her paralyzed arm had fallen behind her and she was lying on her hand; the pillows were in an awkward position. . . . She was wearing a grubby gown and she looked and smelt unwashed . . . she said that bed sores were her worst discomfort . . . but there was no attempt to change her position. At one point during my visit a young student nurse came and sat on a table beside us; she said how bored she was as there was so little to do. . . .

Though fundamentally it deals with the life of a cripple, I would like to reprint here an excerpt from a letter written to me by Miss Michele Gilbert, which she playfully calls "Growing Up Geriatric." Her experience is pertinent in that it describes the treatment many aged patients might expect on a typical geriatric ward:

At the age of sixteen, in 1943, I entered a geriatric ward. There was nowhere else for me, it seemed. An acute attack of rheumatoid arthritis had left me completely incapacitated and in need of permanent care. As there was no one at home to give this the authorities had no alternative. So for twenty-three years the geriatric ward of the Chronic Hospital has been home to me.

During my first night in the hospital I was awakened at 3 A.M. for a wash. I thought I must still be dreaming, but as I peered round the darkened ward I could discern that others were receiving similar treatment. I felt like a character in a Dickens novel, and in the days that followed I came to realize more and more that the social evils which aroused Dickens had not all been left behind in the darkness of the 19th century.

There were twenty-six patients in the ward, not all elderly. It was decorated in the usual institutional dark brown and green, relieved occasionally by dingy cream. Down the center stood a long oak cabinet and this was the principal object of the nurse's loving care. Every afternoon, regardless of staff shortages or patients' immediate needs, that cabinet was polished for at least half an hour. When it was mirror bright it was covered with a clean sheet (sometimes there was a patient who would have been glad of that clean sheet), and under the sheet, for extra protection, was a red blanket.

I witnessed the daily ritual from my bed. I had been put

there on arrival and was told that as I couldn't walk (in actual fact I could) or do anything for myself I would have to stay in bed permanently. The days were monotonous and endless, and the routine unvarying. The rules and regulations in their number and inhumanity might have been devised for a prison. My crime, and that of hundreds like me, was that of being a "young chronic."

After the early wash came the early breakfast—at 6 A.M. This was simply dumped on the locker and there it remained until someone had time to feed it to the helpless patient. Many a time I have fallen asleep while waiting and been rudely awakened by someone anxious to shovel in the congealed bacon and stone-cold tea as rapidly as possible and be done with the job.

It wasn't long before I was in trouble with the authorities because I wanted something to occupy my perfectly normal mind. They suggested I might, as I was so anxious, make an iron holder. I could get a piece of canvas and some wool from the woman who came to the hospital once a week. It amazed them when I made it clear that even this was not enough to satisfy me. I wanted books! And writing materials! I was cluttering up my locker and making the ward look untidy. I even had books on my window sill. What did I want them for? I could only read one at a time couldn't I? Didn't I realize I was in a hospital?

Yes, I realized that. All too well. I realized that this bed and locker were my home and would be for the next fifty years or more. I wanted to take correspondence courses, to learn. This meant more books, as well as papers. On one occasion an irate nurse confiscated everything I needed for my studies and locked them away in a cupboard. It was only my doctor's intervention that got them back for me. When after several years I at last managed to get a typewriter, the comment was: "And where do you think you are going to keep that?"

One day in 1949, just after the coming of the National Health Service [socialized medicine], a group of doctors came round, examining everyone and making notes. We learned that our old Chronic Hospital was to be integrated into a regional hospital group with the local general hospital as its nerve center. . . . The first and most important change that affected me was that I was ordered out of bed. "Whatever do they want to start getting you up for?" grumbled the nurses, as they bundled me into the wheelchair I'd had as a twenty-first birthday present and which had hardly been used. "You've been happy in bed all these years." Fancy. I'd never known that my feelings "all those years" were what is known as "happiness." Did it never occur to them that we could be human enough to feel despair and frustration at the barrenness of our existence?

Then those visiting doctors, appalled to discover how long I had been kept inactive in bed, wanted me to have treatment, and ordered that the newest methods should be tried in my case. "A waste of money," grumbled the nurses, and every excuse was brought for not getting me out of bed, for not giving me that treatment that had been ordered. I had to fight for it, and if I did get it I was deposited back in bed immediately afterwards—the naughty child who must be punished for some tiresome behavior. One day a doctor came round and asked me if I *wanted* to go back to bed so early. After that, my time "up" was extended. For a long time the ward nurse wouldn't speak civilly to me because I had dared to say that I didn't really want to go back to bed at two o'clock in the afternoon.

. . . But this is where we came in. I sit here, the elderly women around me. Many of the evils of the past have been eliminated. I can now go out whenever someone wants to take me, and the staff gets me ready. Visiting times are relaxed from twice a week to twice a day (again, if anyone wants to come). There are more facilities for some kind of mental life. An enlightened matron has provided a cupboard for my things, as well as shutting her eyes to all visible "junk," realizing that this is my "home."

But we are still regimented and ruled by the clock, so that never for a moment do we forget we are "lifers." The slightest deviation from routine seems to set the machinery wrong and panic reigns. Members of the staff are continually bewailing the fact that it's nothing like the old days. Thank goodness it is not. I have revived painful memories that I would rather forget. But so long as there are young people normal in their minds and feelings, lying imprisoned in crippled bodies, in geriatric wards, helpless and hopeless, one must remember, so that the general public are not allowed to forget.

Her description of life on a geriatric ward is corroborated by a letter from a nurse in the Midlands:

I have nursed for the last seven years in a well-known geriatric hospital here. It has a growing reputation, largely due to self-advertisement, for the humanitarian and "new approach" conditions under which the aged patients live. The actual treatment of these helpless old men and women is such that I have taken out an expensive insurance policy in order that I may never find myself a patient there. With the help of another nurse, who feels as I do, I have made a detailed list of the things from which our "confused" old patients suffer most. If you are interested I should like to send you a copy of this. I think you would hardly believe how much roughness, laziness and dirt can go on unchecked in these days.

I asked her to send it. I almost wished I hadn't. Selecting my words with responsible concern, I would describe it as a catalogue of cruelty, callousness, filth, and depersonalization such as I have not read since I was reviewing the reports of the Nuremberg trials—and such as I thought never to read again. I have independent evidence about this nurse's reliability as an observer. I can only suppose that those old people must be longing to die. Why in God's name are we inflicting this treatment on old men and women who have not harmed us?

This nurse offered her list of atrocities to her matron, to the hospital administrator (twice), and to the local press. She told me that they all rejected it. I suppose it would upset too many people, and keeping the truth from the relatives is part of the service offered. You have to be considerate where you can, and where it will be noticed.

# The Question of Pain

*I have been deeply interested in the mechanism of pain and the nature of suffering . . . the only certain fact I have grasped is that . . . severe injury often seems to cause little or no pain. . . .*

—Anonymous doctor

## THE GODS OF LIFE

*With what strife and pains we come into the world we remember not; but 'tis commonly found no easy matter to get out of it.*

—Sir Thomas Browne

Euthanasiasts believe that dying persons are frequently in agony and pain as they go through their final moments. The doctors they quote say that drugs do not always kill pain. On the other hand, other doctors claim that modern medicine can completely eliminate all pain in the terminally ill.

Which is correct?

I believe that the standard pain-killers are not always effective, and that furthermore their side effects—e.g., depression and grogginess—are prodigious. Moreover, the prescription of drugs and administration of dosage in our hospitals is so frequently inept, mistaken, and improper (approximately one-sixth of the time by standard surveys) that the dying patient is lucky indeed to be adequately looked after.

The majority of terminal patients spend their last days either in their own homes or with relatives, where drug control is minimum, or on the wards of ordinary hospitals, where most nurses don't bother too much and where understaffing is a chronic impediment to careful terminal care. The needs of a dying patient on this sort of ward, which is all too often preoccupied with the care of acute and *curable* disease, have a low priority. In such circumstances, relief of his distress may be negligible.

A 1906 study of 500 dying patients found that 18 percent suffered pain or distress of one sort or another. In a 1960 survey of 220 terminally ill patients, it was found that 14 percent suffered from moderate or severe pain. (But, of course, one man's "moderate" may be another's "severe," and then there's always the possibility that patients will minimize their suffering in front of the doctor.) Also, the group most likely to wish for death were those with heart difficulty. Cancer patients suffered severe pain in only about 25 percent of the cases. The group in the greatest pain were those with locomotor difficulty—paraplegics, for example. Locomotor patients had difficulty with their joints and bones. Some had been confined to wheelchairs for years, others had severe arthritis. More than half of these had long-lasting, continuous, and severe pain, which was aggravated by even the gentlest movement. Any disorder of the skeletal system was likely to mean great pain. The stronger drugs gave them virtually no relief.

Contrary to popular belief, sufferers from heart or kidney disease are far more likely than cancer patients to feel distress in the terminal stages. Breathing difficulty, nausea, and vomiting are significantly higher, and this may account for their greater discomfort—pain can frequently be relieved by medication, but nausea and vomiting can be alleviated less than half the time, and breathing difficulty almost never. An English psychiatrist found that he was unable to relieve the pain of 18 percent of his patients, and that of those he was able to help, 37 percent still experienced nausea and 18 percent suffered from shortness of breath. He states:

> The moment of death is not often a crisis of distress for
> the dying person. For most, the suffering is over a while

before they die. Already some of the living functions have failed and full consciousness usually goes early. Before the last moments of life there comes a quieter phase of surrender, the body appears to abdicate peacefully, no longer attempting to survive. Life then slips away so that few are aware of the final advent of their own death.

Other statistics indicate that while only 11 percent of all patients are unconscious in the last week of life, only 6 percent are conscious at the moment of death.

Among victims of cancer, severe and continuous pain is frequently prominent in the final stages of life. But terms can be confusing. If one has cancer of the throat and has to "live" with a tube in it, if breathing and eating are such a struggle that one has no energy for anything else or never gets a good night's sleep, "discomfort" is constant. Exactly when it becomes "pain" is a difficult question. Drugs can do nothing for this sort of distress.

Then there is the mental misery cancer patients feel at the presence of their foul, fungating growth, the slow starvation due to difficulty swallowing, painful and frequent urination, obstructed bowels, incontinence. Take the case of one patient with inoperable cancer of the throat. For months he had been having increasing difficulty swallowing, even liquids, and suffered a great deal of pain. Then the cancer invaded his windpipe and larynx so that breathing and even speaking become difficult. Narcotics were not sufficient to control his pain. When his mind was clear he begged for release from the weeks of misery ahead. Clearly the patient was not functioning as a human being in any social sense. Should he be "released"? With variations in detail, this is the story of about twenty thousand patients each year in Britain and America.

Is there any safe way to mitigate the effects of cancer—perhaps through the use of radium or other treatment approved by the American Medical Association? Here are the words of a dying English surgeon in the *British Medical Journal*: "The surgical part of my case was trivial and painless. But I would not wish on my worst enemy the prolonged hell I have been through with radium infection of my nervous system and pain for over six months." Many doctors concur. The chief of surgery in a Montreal hospital states: "I would beg that if *I* became a 'vegetable' or if I had inoperable cancer that I be allowed to die in peace without any medication other than sedation."

Unfortunately, the powerful pain-killing drugs, such as morphine, often cause depression, shortness of breath, vomiting, and constipation. Further, most pain-killers appear to have a decidedly adverse effect on the ability to sleep, probably because they seriously curtail the patient's ability to dream. (Studies have shown that the hallucinating portion of our sleep is the most revitalizing period.) There is also some deterioration of personality and, for the terminal case particularly, acceleration of dying due to the quietening drugs themselves.

Morphine is an excellent example. Prolonged usage of this drug is acknowledged by everyone to be lethal, particularly when the natural functions have failed, i.e., heart regulation, breathing, salivation. When morphine is no longer effective intravenously because of decreased circulation, it may be injected directly into the heart. Everyone working with this drug knows very well that this is mercy killing in its most basic form. We read and hear constantly that somehow an overdose has been given in a terminal case and someone has died. Might not it be said that the doctor who gives his patient sedatives and narcotics which dull pain but shorten life is, technically at least, practicing euthanasia?

It is true that a very small number of patients have the good fortune to be cared for in hospitals that specialize in easing the last days of terminal illness—for example, the famous St. Christopher's Hospital in London. Such hospitals are specifically organized and administered with the aim of making their patients "fairly comfortable" in their last days; they do not try to cure them when this seems pointless. Most of these hospitals are staffed by dedicated women of some religious order, many of whom are also trained in nursing. These nurses are prepared to provide huge amounts of psychological support in addition to nursing care.

Experience has shown that in the sympathetic and sometimes surprisingly cheerful atmosphere created by these women it is possible for a large proportion of the patients (most of whom have cancer) to be "gentled" along in comparative comfort so that they are able to face death quietly and unafraid. As one nurse has said: "They die like the going out of a candle."

One of St. Christopher's doctors who is a firm opponent of voluntary euthanasia has often declared that in such hospitals no patient would even request euthanasia. This doctor tells how a former head of the Euthanasia Society in Britain once came to investigate St. Christopher's and remarked: "I didn't know you could do it. If all patients died something like this, we could disband the society. . . . I'd like to come and die in your home." Yet the doctor admits that many patients enter the hospital in great pain, and that very occasionally pain can only be controlled by keeping the patient "continually asleep." Is such a continual drugged sleep much different from actual death?

Another St. Christopher's physician has told me privately: "There is no need to go to great lengths to keep them alive— I would not resuscitate or keep them on artificial pacemakers if I was really satisfied that sentient life was extinct." Does "sentient" refer here to *mental* life? I think so. And yet this doctor also is a strong opponent of the euthanasiasts: "I do not think one ever ought to terminate life," she says positively.

Her remarks indicate that she does not consider a skin-muscle-bone system in which the blood is making its appointed rounds as "life." Nor does she believe that breathing necessarily indicates life. "Sentient" means "able to feel"—obviously, patients who can breathe and bleed, but not "feel," are dead in her terms.

The successful work of St. Christopher's Hospital leaves us wondering if doctors and nurses should not be paying more attention to the mechanics of alleviating pain—particularly to the *psycho*-mechanics of it.

Perhaps psychological therapy operating in conjunction with drugs can ease the agony of the terminal patient, as Laszlo and Spencer indicated in *Medical Clinics of North America*:

Fear and anxiety, the patient's need for attention from the family or from the physician, are frequently mistaken for expression of pain. Reassurance and an unhesitating approach in presenting a plan of management to the patient are well-known patient "remedies," and probably a clue to the success of many medical quackeries.

Interestingly, Laszlo and Spencer found that *more than 50 percent* of cancer patients who had received pain-killing drugs for long periods of time could be adequately controlled with placebo medication! This may seem strange until we recall how, at one time or another, we have tossed and turned, finally taken a pill to aid sleep, and gone off immediately, long before the pill could have had a chance to work.

# Dying

PART III

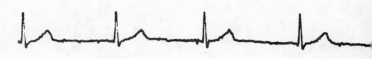

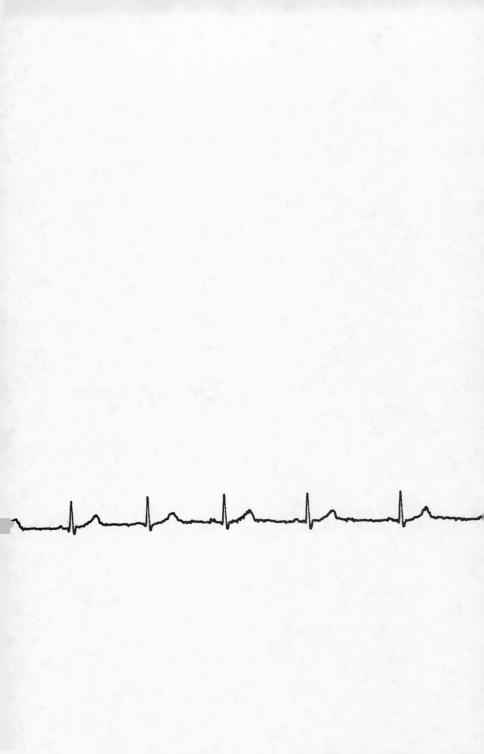

# Prolonging Life or Prolonging Dying?

*I pray you take no more trouble for me. Let me go quietly.*

—George Washington, after repeated bleedings, purgings, and blisterings, common medical practice of his time.

# THE GODS OF LIFE

*. . . cancer of the breast, after six months of horrible suffering.*
*. . . And not a doctor dare have the humanity to put an end to*
*this martyrdom. . . .*

—Berlioz, on the death of his sister

*Vex not his ghost: O, let him pass! He hates him*
*That would upon the wrack of this tough world*
*Stretch him out longer.*

—Shakespeare, *King Lear*, V, iii

An old man with liver disease was deep in a coma and dying.
The attending team of medical experts succeeded in bringing
him out of the coma—so that he could await a fatal
hemorrhage or yet another coma.

A seventy-five-year-old man with rapidly spreading cancer
developed pneumonia, a common death for a terminal patient.
However, antibiotics cured the pneumonia—only to save the
patient for the longer and far more discomforting ordeal of
slowly dying from cancer.

A ninety-year-old woman had a complex of chronic ills and
was mentally inert. She had a heart attack and was placed in
an oxygen tent, put on a pacemaker, fed intravenously, and
given anticoagulatory drugs to help her blood flow more
smoothly. She was given a battery of tests. Within 48 hours
she was dead, bequeathing her family a gigantic hospital bill.

A seventy-six-year-old woman in very feeble health had a
sudden stroke. Her right side was paralyzed and she was
unable to speak. She was put in an ambulance and, sinking

**84**

fast, rushed to a famous teaching hospital. When finally wheeled in, she was, to all intents and purposes, dead. But the young doctors on duty were not dismayed: all the resuscitation equipment the hospital could provide was mobilized, and for eighteen hours the old woman's heart was kept beating and a magnificent artificial respirator did her breathing for her. Mercifully, this determined battle was fought in vain. When later asked what was the point of it, the young doctor gave a facetious but significant reply: although he admitted that even if the woman had lived, she would have been only the shell of a human being, speechless, paralyzed, and demented, he considered it his bounden duty to preserve "life" regardless of any other consideration.

A doctor of sixty-eight was admitted to the hospital with advanced cancer of the stomach, and a subsequent operation revealed that his liver was affected as well. Another operation to remove his stomach followed, and there was evidence of further complications. At last the patient was told of his condition, and, being a doctor, he understood. Despite increasing dosages of drugs, he suffered extreme and constant pain. Ten days after the operation he collapsed with a clot in a lung artery, which was removed in another operation. After a slight recovery, he expressed his appreciation for the skill and good intentions of the surgeon but asked, if he should have another collapse, to be allowed to die peacefully, since the continual pain was more than he wished needlessly to endure. He no longer wanted to "exist" in a hospital as the constant subject for practice operations that would gratify only his surgeon. He even wrote a note to this effect in his case records, and he made sure the staff of the hospital knew his feelings. When he had a heart attack two weeks later, he was resuscitated. The same night his heart stopped again *four times* and each time was artificially restarted. He lingered on for three more weeks, suffering violent vomiting and convulsions. His body was sustained by intravenous feeding, blood transfusions, and various drugs. His heart had stopped so often that his brain cells were dying from oxygen starvation. He was just a piece of mindless wreckage, but nevertheless a whole series of torturous modern techniques were employed to keep him "alive." Preparations were made for using an artificial respirator, but mercifully his heart stopped before it could be used.

After a history of rheumatic heart disease, a patient was admitted to a hospital with a blockage of his heart valves. Open-heart surgery opened the blocked valve, but had to be repeated. Then failing blood pressure brought on a kidney failure. While the doctors were considering the choice between a kidney transplant and putting the patient on an artificial kidney machine, pneumonia set in. Antibiotics were pushed into the patient to treat it, but without success. The doctors then tried a tracheotomy, an operation to open a passage in the throat. But the patient's heart became so weak that even this new opening failed to bring in enough air. Oxygen through nasal tubes was tried, unsuccessfully. Next, a respirator was brought in. Was a machine breathing, or a man?

In New York City a sixty-nine-year-old doctor suffered a stroke and was rushed to the hospital, where he arrived in a deep coma. His heart was still beating, but he had stopped breathing. A tube was inserted into his trachea to make an airway from the respirator to his dormant lungs. Then the respirator commenced to inflate and deflate the lungs with oxygen, keeping the patient alive while doctors analyzed his condition.

It didn't take long to discover that indeed the doctor had no hope of recovery. If artificial respiration were stopped, he would unquestionably "die." Yet the hospital kept the dying man struggling for three days before he was finally allowed to rest. One by one his vital systems broke down irreversibly, yet the doctors continued using the respirator.

In April, 1967, a geriatric nurse wrote in a letter to the *Manchester Guardian*, one of England's leading newspapers:

. . . The stark truth is that all patients dying of old age must now expect, as a matter of routine, to be forced through an additional period, sometimes a long period, of pain and/or acute discomfort before death finally comes. . . . I can think of some examples out of the many I have witnessed . . . one woman dying, aged over one hundred, was given a blood transfusion . . . another very old man, who had been senile for a long time, was kept just alive with artificial feeding and urinary apparatus well after he had become a thing of horror due to advanced gangrene . . . as these two wretched persons were not fully conscious, it could be argued that they were not suffering; but is it civilized or compassionate to lengthen the course of dying in this way?

*The New England Journal of Medicine* reports: "Today's graduate falls heir . . . to the immaculate, modern aseptic skills that can keep a diseased, half-dead, cancerous body alive, by intravenous nourishment and with the magic of penicillin and round-the-clock special nursing. . . ."

Many physicians have asked the question: Does the mere pumping of the vital juices through an inert body constitute life? This question is doubly relevant where medical authorities agree that there is a 100-percent certainty that the patient will soon die, and there is no chance that the patient can be revived.

Even those who vigorously oppose euthanasia are frequently equally opposed to prolonging the vital functions in an obviously "dead" body. Technological progress has made it possible to maintain for a considerable time the appearance of life in a moribund or actually dead patient. The respirator can keep breathing going; the heart function can be similarly supported. Under such circumstances, however, as one doctor puts it: "One is dealing not with a living human being but with a functioning human heart-lung preparation." Such measures hardly seem warranted in the case of a chronically ill person in whom stoppage of the heart or breathing is merely the final outward manifestation of death.

A doctor at the Swedish Society of Surgery believes that we should not regard it as killing by medical means when we refrain from treatment because it does not serve any purpose and is not in the patient's interest. If death has already won, despite our efforts, we must accept the fact. A doctor at a large American clinic takes this position:

> There are too many instances in which patients are suffering excruciating pain, pleading for release, and clearly

beyond saving, yet where they are kept alive indefinitely by means of tubes inserted into their stomachs, or into their veins, or into their rectums . . . all the . . . agents available to us now can keep people suffering for many months. . . .

Drugs and other therapy do not help to alleviate this suffering; as the director of a Stockholm radiation laboratory warns:

> Treatment with large doses of radiation . . . will put the patient at greater disadvantage than may the disease itself. In the individual case it is difficult . . . to judge . . . if, indeed, any type of therapy should be given . . . [further] I will definitely warn the physician not to believe that the patient will be freed from discomfort by giving her large amounts of morphium or similar drugs. . . . In my experience, few patients have a harder time than those which are heavily drugged.

Prolongation of the suffering of the dying may even be illegal, according to one attorney, who asks:

> . . . [Does] keeping alive by artificial means constitute what the law has castigated as experimentation—making guinea pigs out of people? There are a few cases where doctors have prolonged the life of people in coma for months or years—perhaps out of scientific curiosity, without regard to the financial expense to the family. In a Michigan case a family lost everything they had—over $160,000 in medical expenses—for keeping alive a member of the family known to have no chance of rehabilitation.

Today when the dying develop pneumonia, which kills so restfully, they are given penicillin or some other antibiotic.

Should they have heart failure, they are put on a pacemaker or otherwise resuscitated. When they stop breathing, a respirator is called for. Many terminal patients die in a tangle of glass jars, pipettes, tubes with needles in veins, mouth, nostrils, and bladder, and strung up on a cot with ropes, bars, pulleys, and weights, like some kind of barnyard animal. One is reminded of college freshman chemistry laboratories or old horror movies where the mad scientist's laboratory has lights flashing in test tubes. His family can scarcely reach the dying patient through all this junk. And isn't that what we want most at the close, our own families? Should we end in a tangle of wires and tubes, with our loved ones held back by the doctor-technicians?

A doctor describes the following disgusting scene at the bed of a dying man aged ninety-two:

> The surgeon was doing a "cut down" to start an infusion: the nurse with mouth gag and suction apparatus was aspirating secretion from the throat; while the patient, already turned deeply blue, began to have a series of convulsions and died. . . . The picture of that moment remains with me . . . the members of the family who were present, huddled in one corner of the room: They were barred from approaching the bed by oxygen tank, suction apparatus, tubes for suction, catheterization and infusion, as well as by those of the staff at the bedside who had completed the "cut down" and now were attempting artificial aspiration. . . .

Other physicians feel such a situation is appalling. One comments: "Modern methods of resuscitation are decidedly out of place . . . especially when resuscitation would only renew the patient's suffering. . . . The dying ought to be allowed to depart in peace." And John J. Farrell, M.D., had this to say in an address to the American College of Surgeons:

In our pursuit of the scientific aspects of medicine, the art of medicine has sometimes unwittingly and unjustifiably suffered. We have, on occasions, been so concerned with the "right of all men to live" that we are in danger of forgetting that it is appointed for all men once to die. . . . The last words, if the patient has not been comatose for the past forty-eight hours, are lost behind an oxygen mask.

American hospitals, according to one New York doctor, have put barriers of technological apparatus between the patient and the physician, and between the patient and the family. An assistant director of social services at another New York City hospital concurs:

Any visitor to an intensive care unit in a medical institution would be appalled—typewriters go, bells ring, lights light, and the whole milieu is one of crisis and very little human contact. At the time when the patient is most critically ill, the support and visits of his family, friends, or relatives is severely curtailed and the closest thing to him is a monitoring machine.

In former times most people approached the end of life in the privacy of their homes with their family to attend them and with only a minimum of medicine to prolong life. Our big metropolitan hospitals have provided care and alleviation for those in pain, but they have also made dying an undignified ordeal.

An anonymous widow reports:

> He came out of surgery alive. He had not succumbed to this first ordeal. Could I let my tears fall now and then rush in to hug him? Could I tell him there would never be an end to us? Could I tell him he had won this fight against all odds, that he was brave and fine? . . . But I left, as *they* told me to. . . .

Another says that no one thought her husband could survive a "necessary" second operation, but he was given one anyway—a patient so weak is in no condition to oppose anything. The hospital formula at such times is a code language: "The patient is holding his own."

One afternoon she arrived at the hospital and found that her husband had been taken to surgery. "There was need for some repair," said the nurse. It turned out that it had been necessary to operate without anesthetic, presumably because it would be too "dangerous" for the patient. "There is no use going to see the patient," said the doctor. "He will not know you, and now that the operation is over we are going to give him some sedatives."

> I knew that I must see him . . . now, if we were nearing the end of our time together, I must memorize every detail of this scene. . . . They had put the metal bedsides up so that he would not fall out. His eyes and face were wild and he was shouting, though no one could understand him. The long thin arms were all bruised, red and blue. I choked with anguish and horror. . . .

For three savage days and nights the dying man drowned in his delirium, crying out at phantoms, tortured by his wild imagination. Then, after a brief respite, he went into a deep coma:

> The glaring merciless rays from a powerful ceiling light displayed what was a human form, now portrayed in ghastly hue, in hunched position, with two tubes one in each nostril, eyes half open, breathing a noise of horror, while the oxygen tank at one side bubbled, bubbled merrily, and the nurse stood counting heartbeat and pulse. . . . I froze to my depths. . . .

The classic deathbed scene, with its loving partings and solemn last words, is now part of history. In its place is a drugged, unconscious patient full of tubes for breathing, eating, and elimination, a subhuman object for manipulation by the medical technicians. Who can remain unhorrified hearing a doctor on a terminal ward remark that he must "go water the vegetables"?

In the opinion of some doctors:

> One of the greatest comforts for the dying is to be left at home. General hospitals are unhappily places where house staff probe and test, where nurses though not unkind are indifferent, where in brief, the "crock" is a second class citizen. To be in one's own bed, to have quiet and good light, comfortable temperature, books, tasteful food and drink served at reasonable times, this is the final boon a family can give their loved one. It is sometimes impossible, but with the help of friends, visiting nurses, perhaps a night nurse, it can often be managed. Professional nursing

is expensive but, if costs must be considered, it can be balanced against the useless X-rays and laboratory procedures and the other extras one finds on hospital bills.

And a story is told of the case of a woman who died in the "Hollywood" way. At seventy-eight she had had a minor cancer removed, only for it to recur elsewhere. Then she had a stroke, lost the power of speech, and was paralyzed on one side. One vein after another succumbed to the trauma of intravenous feeding, and she was fed through a tube in her nose. Her good arm and leg had to be restrained, or the tube would come out. It was not long before the old woman made it clear that she preferred to die in peace, free of restraint, and free of the tubes. At last her doctor consented to her hand-signal request that the tube be removed. At the same time she was untied, and all other evidences of extraordinary help taken away. Her nurse then went to work to make her as attractive and comfortable as possible, while her doctor telephoned her family and minister.

The changed situation was explained while the patient nodded approval. Moderate sedation and pain-killers were provided as she began turning blue.

> The minister gave a brief and beautiful prayer, and then one by one the family members . . . sat beside the patient's bed and each expressed love, and reminded the old woman briefly of some treasured memory. The husband was last. He took his place and leaned close to whisper. The patient smiled, sighed briefly, and died.

Most people are not so lucky. Today people are dying more like manipulated objects rather than as masters of their fates.

The doctors have become the technological masters. When you enter their hospitals for the last time, it will be *they* who decide how and when you shall die, not you or your family.

The technology brought into play to cheat death staggers the imagination. Devices mechanical, chemical, and surgical are breathtaking in their array and scope. Who can deny their power? They intimidate by their very existence. And yet, interestingly enough, these gadgets actually hasten the death of the *personality*, that is, conscious decision and integrity, self-possession. A patient dominated by such technology, by the hospital, and by the entire medical profession is in no condition to take issue with them in his weakened state. Terminal cases in sloppy slippers, robes, and pajamas are not in a position to upstage doctors. The patient is the *object*, not the *prime mover* in this situation. If he is poor or otherwise unimportant, he will be experimented upon. If he is well-to-do, he will be kept clinically and biologically "alive" long after he has become personally dead in every meaningful sense. Doctors have been known to keep patients "alive" on a pacemaker for weeks—"for teaching purposes."

People have noted this. They are asking for doctors who won't make them "go through what father did" or live on a machine "like Aunt Nora." Today they consider more frequently the means of *avoiding* the "help" of doctors.

Dr. David Karnofsky of the Sloan-Kettering Institute, in a 1961 speech, told the American Cancer Society of a patient who had a cancer of the large bowel. After making an artificial opening into the colon which was unsuccessful, X-rays were used. Then radioactive phosphorus checked abdominal fluids, and an antibiotic halted bronchopneumonia. Transfer of the cancer to the liver quickly ended the functions of that organ despite all attempts at interference. When the patient finally went, his dying had been prolonged by nine months. Was it ethical to add this time to his dying? How did it benefit the patient to be worked over, stupefied as a rag doll? Who benefited from this, outside of the practicing doctors?

When Shakespeare wrote "To be or not to be, that is the question," he was quite correct. At that time it was the *only* question. But today, due to the giant strides of modern medical technology, it is very far from being the only question. Men can be and yet not be. They can function in one way and be lost in another. The line between life and death has become blurred. An article in the *British Medical Journal* describes the problem as due partly to medical progress in keeping people alive, rather than preventing them from dying; and that for many of them life holds out no prospects for a worthwhile existence, for large numbers have reached an age and condition in which their only prospect is mental or physical suffering.

What we term "extraordinary support" falls roughly into the following distinctions:

1. Artificial respirators to promote breathing.
2. Heart massage, use of the pacemaker or other machines for stimulation of the heart muscle.
3. Kidney machine to replace worn-out kidneys.
4. Transplant of vital organs.
5. Prolonged medication (i.e., to create favorable blood pressure).
6. Prolonged intravenous feeding.

It is now possible to keep people "alive" for many years though they are unconscious or in a coma. But even a short period of coma can result in very damaged mental faculties. Is a man alive merely because his body creates wastes and his blood is circulating? Are reflexes, circulation, and respiration ends in themselves? Does the personality count for nothing? As a doctor says: "It is now possible to keep a dying person 'alive' almost indefinitely, and as medical tradition is such that doctors are frightened of an impairment of a patient's right to live, accordingly people are kept alive against all good sense."

Because of a vastly increased ability to cushion the discomforting effects of *symptoms*, we are living longer with diseases which were formerly rapidly fatal. Today persons with such long-term diseases are frequently in and out of hospitals long before the final ending. Their lives are now being technically maintained by complex new equipment. Changes in anesthetic and surgical techniques also permit a far greater number of formerly hazardous operations—particularly in large city hospitals and teaching hospitals. Extensive heart surgery and kidney transplants have become commonplace, although the chances of recovery are, thus far, negligible.

The new machinery has somewhat complicated the question of deciding when a person is dead. There has been a marked increase in the use of "heroic" measures, particularly among the younger and more adventurous doctors. This life-prolonging equipment gives the doctor somewhat greater control over the patient's existence, but it also poses some rather difficult questions. When recovery is no longer possible, is it life that is being prolonged, or is it merely death? Life is, after all, something more than merely being able to brush one's teeth in the morning, and many of the "machine patients" are unable to do even that.

Both the Roman Catholic Church and Jewish Law are opposed to euthanasia, but both sanction the withdrawal of artificial factors which merely delay the death of an individual who is obviously dying. Dr. Bruno Haid, chief of the anesthesia section of the surgical clinic at the University of Innsbruck in Austria, raised this question with Pope Pius XII while attending the International Congress of Anesthesiologists in Rome in 1957:

> Sometimes it happens that there is no hope for a patient and that he lingers for days, kept alive only by artificial respiration. In such cases there is sometimes doubt that the patient is truly living—is there a right, then, or even an obligation to use modern apparatus for artificial respiration, even if the case is considered hopeless? May one legitimately remove artificial respiration apparatus, with certain death following, when after several days the state of deep unconsciousness does not improve? When can an individual whose circulation depends entirely on artificial respiration be considered dead?

The Pope replied that artificial respiration was not obligatory, and that machinery could be disconnected without considering this act to be euthanasia. Explicitly: "Human life continues for as long as its vital functions . . . manifest themselves spontaneously without the help of artificial processes."

No religion requires that doctors keep alive utterly helpless heart and lung systems which cannot independently support a conscious human being. It appears somewhat curious then that so much doctoring, hospital space, and equipment are often devoted to just this activity, to the detriment of those who might be said to be more fully "alive." The British medical journal *Lancet* has pointed out: "If the average length of a patient's stay in a hospital is two weeks, a bed in that hospital occupied for a year could have been used by 26 other patients. . . . In a country without a surplus of hospital beds, an irrevocably unconscious patient may sometimes be kept alive at the cost of other people's lives."

We need to reexamine our whole definition of death and dying. Margaret Mead, the famed socio-anthropologist, has said in *Childhood in Contemporary Cultures*:

> I believe that in each age it is appropriate to rethink the responsibilities which each individual carries in regard to his own life and the life of others. In this present age we have reached a crisis because medical advances have outdistanced our expected forms of behavior.

Luis Kutner, an attorney who is also the originator of World Habeas Corpus and a Nobel Prize nominee, feels that:

> Advancing medical technology is coming face-to-face with a complete reorganization of our former definitions of "aliveness." This confrontation promises to become even more acute as life is produced by laboratory means or genes are controlled. . . . Perhaps a better approach to this problem might be to define what constitutes death. . . .

Several years ago Dr. Kenneth O. A. Vickery made headlines by saying at a convention of the Royal Society of Health in England that geriatric patients were overloading hospital and welfare services in England. He said that medicine must face squarely the issue of "medicated survival":

> . . . in a community which can no longer adequately nurse all its chronic sick and where beds are so blocked by the aged that younger people requiring surgical and medical treatment cannot be admitted, we can no longer avoid the issue of medicated survival, which as so successfully manifested in the current medical practice is surely one of the cruelest hazards to which we can be subjected.

Dr. Vickery said that he had deliberately spoken on the "grim and depressing" aspects of this problem to draw attention to its urgency. Thirteen percent of Britain's population are now retired persons, and that figure is rising. Vickery was quoted as saying:

> Standards remain such that once a patient is lucky enough to secure a hospital bed, he becomes eligible for the ultimate in medical and nursing care, including heroic resuscitation to snatch him from the jaws of death, and the latest in modern medication to keep pneumonia at bay. It is submitted that the time has come for a minimum age to be agreed beyond which medical and nursing staff may be relieved of the prevailing obligation "officiously to keep alive" and confine their ministrations to symptomatic relief and good nursing.

An eighty-three-year-old official of England's Federation of Old Age Pensioners was somewhat in agreement. He commented, "It's not right to bring an old person back to life when he is nearly dead. When a person comes near to the time of dying, he should be left to die. It is a natural thing that when one gets old, death doesn't mean much. If I suddenly became ill, and thought I would not get better, I would like to be left to die peacefully."

# To Be or Not to Be:
## Toward a New
## Definition of Death

*Life is only sweet if you can see a sunset or smell a flower.*

—Anonymous

Few people are aware of the essential limitations of the new technology. Nature has set unappealable limits. After a certain period of oxygen starvation, for example, the brain will quickly disintegrate, leaving the physician holding the wrists of a "vegetable" which is human only in appearance.

Not long ago, a three-year-old girl was on an operating table when an obstruction formed in the air line which was bringing her oxygen. For five minutes, maybe six, she received no oxygen. Without warning, her little heart stopped beating. What had started as the routine repair of a cleft palate had become a tragedy.

A hurried call was put through for the staff anesthesiologist, who raced to clear the vital airway by directing the surgeon to open the girl's chest. The sharp scalpel cut between the ribs on the side of the chest; rubber-gloved hands pulled the ribs apart and reached into the chest to take hold of the heart. Compressing the heart between palm and fingers, the physician squeezed blood into the dormant arteries. At last the heart fluttered, then stopped again, and finally resumed its work. A respirator was wheeled into place to keep that rekindled flame going. Soon the heart beat strongly on its own. The lungs took in air, and it seemed as if modern technology had won again.

But hours, weeks, and finally months passed—and the little girl did not regain consciousness. Her heart beat, she breathed, but the brightness of her mind had been snuffed like a candle in a high wind. During the terrible minutes when her heart stopped, no oxygen had reached her brain. The doctors failed to restore circulation within the minimum time required by nature. At first a few brain cells died. Then more and more. By the time the frantic doctors brought more oxygen to her brain, all her mental faculties had perished. Her brain was dead. And brains do not revive.

That was four years ago. The little girl will never regain consciousness. She is occupying a hospital bed that could serve twenty-six patients each year. She is using valuable equipment that might salvage more authentically human lives.

The cerebral cortex of a boy of twenty was shattered in an auto accident four years ago. All thought and feeling have been erased from his once strong body and he hasn't moved a muscle since. The doctors say he is in "excellent health" although he feels nothing, inside or outside. Once a strong blond youth, he now looks like a dark-haired, baby-faced boy of ten years. He is fed through a nasal tube. But he is not in pain. Is he dead or alive?

When heart and lungs pause, oxygen is no longer pumped to the brain. An adult's brain can stand up to five minutes of oxygen starvation without extensive destruction of cells; a child's may withstand up to ten minutes. Since the heart can sometimes be made to resume beating after as much as ten minutes of silence, it is often possible to restore the appearance of life only to find that the patient's brain no longer exists. A doctor at a midwest university states: "I have seen patients with brain-stem failure, with dilated fixed pupils, decerebrate rigidity, and no spontaneous breathing, who have had a tracheostomy and were assisted with a mechanical respirator. With fluids, electrolytes, and good nursing, the essentially isolated heart in such a patient can sometimes be kept beating for a week." An anesthesiologist at a New England hospital has said: "Inevitably . . . more and more patients will accumulate in hospitals in the land, near misses, people who can be kept alive only by extraordinary means, in whom there is no hope of recovery of consciousness, let alone hope of recovery to a functioning existence." He reminds us that the cost of keeping a hopelessly injured patient alive for a year is about $30,000.

Of two hundred patients who died in the Intensive Care Unit of the Massachusetts General Hospital between 1961 and 1969, about 20 percent were unconscious for a long period before their death and it was thought their brains would be useless even in the unlikely event that they did revive. They were, to all intents and purposes, vegetables, unsalvageable as human beings.

A doctor comments: "Certainly the human spirit that emerges in man's unique individuality is the product of his brain, not his heart. . . . Medical lore has enthroned the heart through the ages as the sacred chalice of life's blood." The heart originally received this honor from the ancient Chinese physicians, and its preeminence was magnified by modern discoveries about circulation. In former times the heart was considered *the* most central organ in the body, the most important for the continuation of life. Until the recent past, it was accurate enough to consider the heart as the demarcation line between life and death because all parts of the body "died" in close temporal proximity. If any one system in the body necessary to its existence failed, the others were sure to fail within five minutes. This meant that if the heart stopped, the other vital systems would also stop soon after. Similarly with the brain system, the lungs, and so on—the loss of any one meant death.

This is no longer true. Today the heart may stop and start many times before the individual actually dies. The new technology can revive a heart many times. Electrical devices (e.g., the pacemaker), heart massage, the use of oxygen under pressure, and other methods have served to "bring back to life" those who formerly would have been considered officially dead. Now a man's lungs may die, but not his brain. A man's brain may die, but not his heart. And so on. The picture is confused.

If the brain dies, the surviving body exists in a vegetable state; yet legally this vegetable is a live human being. The following case will serve to illustrate some of the difficulties involved.

A thirty-two-year-old man was admitted to a British hospital suffering from fractures of the skull and extensive brain damage received in a barroom brawl. About fourteen hours later, he stopped breathing. At this point his wife's consent was sought and granted for removing one of his kidneys for transplanting to a man dying of kidney disease. Artificial respiration by machine was started on the patient and was continued for twenty-four hours until the kidney was transplanted. The respirator was then turned off. Note that the patient did not breathe or circulate blood spontaneously.

At the inquest a pathologist stated that the man had died from the brain damage and that, therefore, the removal of his kidney came after death. The coroner in the case, however, believed that the patient's attachment to the machine made his body technically "alive" although his brain had died. Was the man alive or dead when the kidney was removed? Because he was on a respirator, his lungs were "breathing" and his blood was circulating. Does this constitute "life"? The jury returned a verdict of manslaughter against the patient's assailant.

The definition of death has become very complex. If loss of brain functions constitutes death, what about the thousands of persons in mental institutions who are no longer functioning mentally? Are they dead? Alternately, if a person is dead when respiration ceases, what about those of sound mind who are living inside iron lungs which do their breathing for them? Should they be considered "dead"? If death comes when the heart stops beating, what about those who are revived? When their hearts stopped beating, did their estates automatically pass to their heirs? Were their wives or husbands free to marry again in the interim?

Today we know more about death than we used to. We know, for example, that there is probably no such thing as "the instant of death." Like life, death is a *process,* not a moment. Certain tissues can be preserved for months when removed from human patients, and when reimplanted, they live and function again. A human heart can be revived as late as one-half hour after it has been deprived of its blood supply and has been technically dead. A leg muscle can be revived ten hours after "death." The nails, hair, and parts of the skin continue to grow for days after "death."

The brain is perhaps the most vulnerable part of the body.

If deprived of oxygenated blood, for as little as three to five minutes, irreversible damage begins. In the rare event that such a victim is saved, his heart, kidneys, and liver may function for years even while his brain is, to all purposes, quite dead. Modern medicine faces this particular problem constantly. Consequently, there is a move in some medical circles to redefine death.

Medical dictionaries define death as the absence of a heartbeat and lack of breathing, and this is the guideline in the courts. Law dictionaries define death as a total stoppage of the circulation of the blood and the ceasing of the vital functions dependent on this circulation. However, they also grant that "death" may be defined by *physicians*. Therefore, since the courts regard the general opinion among physicians to be the determining factor in defining death, all the medical profession need do to change the law is to *change their own definition of death*. The matter rests with them.

Perhaps the strongest possibility for a new definition lies in the petition of the Ad Hoc Committee of the Harvard Medical School that a flat EEG tracing become the new definition of death. The EEG, or electroencephalograph, is a device which measures electrical impulses emanating from the brain—otherwise known as "brain waves." Impulses from the brain appear as wavy lines on the EEG screen. If the line is flat for any reasonable length of time, the brain will not revive.

The brain develops very early in the life of the human being. EEG readings have been taken from the heads of aborted embryos only forty days old and half an inch long.

Embryo brains older than forty-five days have shown response to drugs, response to lack of oxygen, and normal sleep patterns. Thus, in the very earliest stages of life, the pattern of the brain is established. And its EEG pattern, in every case, is individual and unique. This is quite different from the heart/blood circulatory system, which is relatively similar in all people.

It can usually be determined fairly readily whether or not a patient's brain is irretrievably damaged, and whether consciousness will ever return. In such a case the electroencephalograph will usually show that the cerebral cortex has been destroyed, and this can easily be confirmed via air encephalography. In such cases, the human being is reduced to those activities that can be supported by the rear portion of the brain. To keep such a fragmentary creature alive requires the services of a skilled team of doctors and nurses, working in masks to forestall lung infection, treating by bronchoscopic suction and antibiotics if necessary, and feeding the patient artificially. Not only must this nursing care be very extensive, but the full resources of the laboratory must be called upon for biochemical and bacteriological tests.

This type of unconscious state is all the more disturbing when the patient retains an appearance of relative health, as opposed to the type of unconsciousness which is progressively deteriorating. Pink cheeks and gentle breathing give an appearance of natural sleep, from which an awakening may be expected in time, as with Sleeping Beauty. Worse still, the patient's eyes may open from time to time, and follow someone moving around the bed with an unseeing gaze. It is difficult not to accept those eyes as being connected to a conscious mind. Relatives who cannot comprehend the irreversibility of severe brain damage often refuse to abandon hope and think it a betrayal of trust for the doctor to do so.

The EEG unit at Massachusetts General Hospital has collected the records of more than fifty long-term unconscious respirator patients, three of whom have survived, but each with catastrophic disability of their nervous system. One such patient has "lived" over a year in this zombie state, a triumph of protoplasmic resuscitation. Dr. Robert Schwab, head of the department, has accepted the responsibility—with the support of his colleagues—for the determination by EEG of death over fifteen times in the last three years. And patients' families have been generally relieved to have cases handled in this fashion.

The Ad Hoc Committee would judge irreversible coma—and thus the death of the brain—by the following criteria:

1. *Lack of reception and reflex*—even the most intensely painful stimulus evokes no reaction from the patient; not a groan, the withdrawal of a limb, or the quickening of breathing.

2. *Lack of movement or breathing*—after watching the patient for one hour or more, physicians note no spontaneous muscle movements of any kind, no breathing, or response to stimuli.

3. *Total absence of reflexes*—including lack of response by the pupil of the eyes to direct light.

4. *Flat EEG.*

5. *All of the above have the same status twenty-four hours later.*

6. The validity of the above scheme as a measure of irreversible brain damage depends on two conditions:

   *a.* body temperature above ninety degrees.

   *b.* no presence in the body system of barbiturates or other depressants.

The Ad Hoc Committee's position is that satisfaction of all the above conditions will justify turning off respirators and other equipment that is keeping the patient "alive."

Along the same lines, the French Academy of Medicine has voted unanimously to accept brain death as definitive, and specified a negative EEG reading of forty-eight hours.

It must be recognized, however, that apparent EEG silence may ensue for reasons other than brain death. After severe trauma, during heart attacks, or in postoperative states, a patient may indeed register a relatively flat EEG. Patients under freezing anesthesia who are undergoing heart surgery, where they are on blood circulation equipment and there is still severe loss of blood, where the heart has lost its smooth rhythm and becomes awkward, may show loss of brain waves for brief periods. Dr. Hannibal Hamlin has reported in the *Journal of the American Medical Association* a case in which a teen-age girl was comatose and without brain waves for up to *three days*, and yet recovered, virtually spontaneously. Therefore, if a patient is still breathing, and his heart is still pumping, the average doctor would probably feel decidedly uneasy about signing a death certificate, regardless of the activity or inactivity of the brain.

Another case was reported by Drs. Tentler, Sadove, Becka, and Taylor in a 1957 article in the *Journal of the American Medical Association*, "Electroencephalographic Evidence of

Cortical 'Death' Followed for Full Recovery." Their report was based on findings from a study made at the Veterans Hospital at Hines, Illinois.

A twenty-four-year-old man was brought into the hospital with fractures of his vertebrae after a gunshot wound. His symptoms were paraplegic and spastic, and he was incontinent. He had suffered severe cord trauma and evidenced liquefaction of the spinal cord. During a variety of medical procedures too involved to detail here, the patient suffered three severe brain hemorrhages, the longest lasting nineteen and one-half minutes. Each time, the complete absence of cortical rhythm was shown as a flat tracing on the attached electroencephalogram. Such a prolonged loss of cortical activity ordinarily signals severe brain anemia and irreversible damage. More than five minutes of such a condition will usually destroy a brain beyond repair. Yet, contrary to this expectation, no psychological, neurological, or general behavioral impairment was evident.

Another problem in establishing a flat EEG as the criterion of death is that the hyperfast *beta* brain wave, which resembles the flat EEG, may sometimes emanate from comatose patients.

How are we to resolve problems such as these? Just what will be the new definition of death?

# To Euthanatize or
# Not to Euthanatize

*When a tortured man asks, "For God's sake, doctor, let me die,"
we have yet to find the answer as to whether to comply is for
God's sake, the patient's sake, our own, or possibly all three. . . .*

—Dr. Edgar E. Filbey, England

## THE GODS OF LIFE

*If one death is accompanied by torture, and the other is simple
and easy, why not snatch the latter?*

—Seneca

*. . . life, physical life, is not sacrosanct. That is not a Christian
idea at all; for if it were, then the martyrs erred.*

—Archbishop Temple, Anglican Church

It has been said that the first known request for euthanasia
was that of King Saul in 1013 B.C. When the Philistines had
killed his sons and were rapidly destroying what remained of
his army, Saul begged his adjutant: "Draw your sword and
kill me; it would be better for me to die by your hand than
for the Philistines to come upon me and slaughter me." His
officer refused, however, and Saul was forced to commit suicide: "Then Saul took his own sword and fell upon it and
killed himself among the bodies of his own men." So voluntary
euthanasia has a very ancient history on the battlefield.

Before the Christian era in Europe, voluntary euthanasia
("easy death") was considered a reasonable practice. Pythag-
oras, the famed mathematician, endorsed it in the sixth century B.C. So did Plato and Aristotle. Augustus prayed for it.
Sophocles was another enthusiastic voluntary euthanasiast,
and Zeno, founder of the Stoic school, is said to have taken
his life after he wrenched a finger. Death was considered to
be a morally neutral pursuit, sometimes even preferable to
life.

Seneca, in what is probably the most eloquent dissertation on the subject, wrote:

> Against all the injuries of life I have the refuge of death. If I can choose between a death of torture and one that is simple and easy, why should I not select the latter? As I choose the ship in which I sail and the house which I shall inhabit, so will I choose the death by which I leave life. . . . Why should I endure the agony of disease . . . when I can emancipate myself from all torments? . . . I will not relinquish old age if it leaves my better part intact. But if it begins to shake my hand, if it destroys its faculties one by one, if it leaves me not life but breath, I will depart from the putrid or tottering edifice. If I know that I must suffer without hope of relief I will depart not through fear of the pain itself but because it prevents all for which I would live.

Many of the Stoics were enthusiastic about suicide when life became miserable. King Ptolemy had to forbid Hegesias the Cyreniac from lecturing, for too many in his audience were killing themselves after listening to him! The younger Pliny recommended that the right to die when one pleased was "God's best gift to men among the sufferings of life." Pliny described a poet who starved himself to death voluntarily: "Bad health was the cause. He developed an incurable tumor, and wearying of it, he betook himself to death with irrevocable firmness."

On Kos, the island birthplace of Hippocrates, it was customary for old men to drink the hemlock together. And according to the medical historian Sigerist, it was quite common for doctors to poison their patients if they were dying painfully. Theophrastus, in his book on the history of plants, wrote of potions of hemlock specifically improvised for this purpose. Thus, an acceptance of, even admiration for, euthanasia under special circumstances was the prevalent attitude in ancient Greece and Rome.

For the first two centuries after Christ this attitude prevailed. But from its Judaic and Hellenist sources Christianity gradually developed an intransigence on the subject which eventually led to the complete prohibition of voluntary euthanasia. The Renaissance brought no changes in orthodox attitudes, but it did permit radical opinion to emerge after centuries of repression. Sir Thomas More, Francis Bacon, John Donne, Montaigne, and later Rousseau, David Hume, and Voltaire were among those who took up the cudgel for compassionate euthanasia.

Jonathan Swift, that literary giant of the eighteenth century, was probably the most famous example of his times of the need for euthanasia. He died a degrading and horrifying death; his mind literally crumbled to pieces. It took him eight years to die as his brain rotted. Every year on his birthday, so long as he could see, he read aloud from the third chapter of Job: "And Job spoke, and said, let the day perish when I was born and the night in which it was said, 'There is a man-child conceived.' " The pain in his eyes was so fierce that it sometimes took five men to hold him down to keep him from ripping them out with his own fingers. For his final three years he sat and drooled like a baby. Knives had to be kept entirely out of his reach so he would not commit suicide. When the end finally came, his convulsions lasted a day and a half and were frightening to behold. In every sense Swift's death was degrading to both himself and all those who knew and revered him. Should any man be permitted to fall into such physical ruin and spiritual annihilation? Swift wrote to his niece fully five years before his finish: "I am so stupified and confused that I cannot even express the mortification I am under both of body and soul."

Nietzsche, whose health was bad, several times took overdoses of chloral in the hope that he would die. Freud, who had condemned *thanatos*, the death instinct, as immature, asked for a lethal injection to end his suffering from cancer of the jaw and was obliged by his physician.

Probably the first euthanasia debate of the modern era took place in the 1870s in England, when L. A. Tollemache published "The New Cure for Incurables" in the *Fortnightly Review* in support of S. D. Williams' position in favor of voluntary euthanasia. Tollemache was bitterly criticized by *The Spectator*, and the battle was engaged. It is still going on.

Among the Anglo-American nations, the euthanasiasts have had their greatest success in Britain. In 1936, some leading English doctors, including a former president of the Royal College of Physicians and Surgeons, tried to introduce a bill in Parliament that would legalize *voluntary* euthanasia in certain heavily proscribed circumstances. The bill was defeated, but with the energetic support of the Euthanasia Society the debate started a trend in public opinion which has been expanding constantly ever since. The euthanasiasts managed to introduce another bill into the House of Lords in 1950. Such controversy was engendered, however, that it was never voted on.

In the summer of 1961 the Suicide Bill was passed by Parliament without opposition, a significant indication of the current trend of opinion. But although the bill removed suicide from the list of criminal offenses, it remained an offense to aid, counsel, or procure an act of self-destruction, an offense which in England carries a maximum penalty of fourteen years in prison. The success of this bill is particularly significant when we consider that the assumed motive for about 18 percent of all London suicides is physical illness.

A later bill to legalize euthanasia was defeated 61–40 in the House of Lords in 1969. On April 7, 1970, Laborite Dr. Hugh Gray submitted another proposal in the House of Commons "to make lawful administration of euthanasia at the request of the patient." This bill was shouted down.

Admittedly, it is not likely that such a bill will prove acceptable very soon—but each year it is *more* acceptable than it was previously. And the euthanasia lobby in Britain is influential and growing.

The following describes a recent, and perhaps important, case in the United States:

*The New York Times*, Sunday, June 24, 1973.

**Jersey Slayer of Paralyzed Brother in Hospital Called a Hero and a Villain by Shore Neighbors.**

Neptune, N. J., June 23—"I don't think he should ever serve a day in jail," said a policeman.

"Nobody has the right to take another person's life, no matter what the circumstances," said a woman shopper.

"It seems to me that fella had a lot of courage, and I guess maybe a lot of love," said an elderly man. "I don't know if I could do such a thing."

Opinions varied, but many people in Monmouth County had them today about 23-year-old Lester Zygmaniak's apparent mercy killing of his paralyzed brother, George, 26, in the intensive care unit of the Jersey Shore Medical Center here.

George, according to a source close to the case, had begged to be killed after being paralyzed from the neck down in a motorcycle accident last Sunday on his family's 18-acre rural property in Millstone Township in western Monmouth County . . . one of the best-known criminal lawyers in the state, who has been retained by the family, said today that euthanasia had never been used successfully as a defense in a murder case in New Jersey.

(Lester Zygmaniak was tried and found not guilty by reason of insanity.)

As of this writing the support for voluntary euthanasia in the United States does not appear very strong. Bills to legalize euthanasia introduced into the legislatures of Nebraska in 1935 and New York in the last several decades have always failed. A bill simpler than the English bill was introduced in the New York legislature in 1947, sponsored by about 6 percent of the New York medical profession, but was defeated.

The cause of euthanasia was probably severely retarded by

the Nazis, who promoted it "eugenically" during World War II. Under the Nazi program *millions* of the "unfit" were put to death. German doctors were unduly eager to receive specified numbers of "unfits" to use in "medical" experiments. Of course, since these people were considered technically inferior, it is not clear how valuable their reactions were to "science."

The Nazi policy of euthanasia was first introduced by a secret order from Adolf Hitler on September 1, 1939. At first it was confined to Germans, then extended to include foreigners. The Reich Committee for Research on Hereditary Diseases and Constitutional Susceptibility to Severe Diseases originally dealt only with children up to age three; but this limit was later raised successively to eight, twelve, sixteen, and seventeen years of age. It is interesting to note the Nazi rationale for extending the criteria for euthanasia candidates so that they could do away with the aged, the chronically ill, the "useless eaters," and the political opposition: ". . . if it is right to take the life of useless and incurable persons, as suggested in the United States and England, then it is right to take the lives of persons who are destined to die for political reasons. . . ."

It must be noted further that the original Nazi pitch to the public was made on behalf of the distressingly ill and incurable, as described by an article on "Medical Science under Dictatorship" (*New England Journal of Medicine,* 1949) which states:

> Adults were propagandized by motion pictures . . . one
> film depicted the life history of a woman suffering from

multiple sclerosis; in it her husband, a doctor, finally
kills her to the accompaniment of soft piano music rendered
by a sympathetic colleague in an adjoining room. Acceptance of this ideology was implanted even in the children. . . . This attitude concerned itself in the early stages
merely with the severely and chronically sick. Gradually
the sphere of those to be included in this category was
enlarged. . . .

Despite this tainted connection to Nazi policies, voluntary
euthanasia has a great many more adherents today than it did
in the thirties. This may be because contemporary societies
are more "permissive," or because there are a lot more
people being kept artificially alive. In any case, it is a topic
discussed much more openly than it was in 1934. And there
are a great many countries where it is more or less tolerated.

In Switzerland, euthanasia is not regarded as murder if the
motive is to effect a compassionate release from incurable
suffering. Under Swiss law, a surgeon may not cut into a dying
patient, and Swiss penal code exempts physicians for actions
performed in discharge of professional duty. The Swiss penal
code distinguishes between killing with malice and killing with
good intent. "Homicide on request" is also a mitigating circumstance. Thus far there have been no noticeable abuses,
although the Swiss were forewarned that passage of the bill
was "the thin edge of the wedge."

In Italy, euthanasia is a crime only if the victim is under
eighteen years of age, retarded, or unduly intimidated. Tolerant laws exist also in the Netherlands, Denmark, Yugoslavia,
and even Catholic Spain. In Germany and Norway, a com-

passionate motive and/or "homicide upon request" operates to reduce the "crime's" penalty. Uruguayan law completely excuses euthanasia, and passive euthanasia is legal in Sweden. Because there is no specific provision for euthanasia in Anglo-American law, it is accounted either suicide when performed by the patient, or murder when performed by another.

The word "euthanasia," derived from the Greek, originally meant a pleasant or easy death. Another modern descriptive term is "mercy killing." Euthanasia societies often refer to it as "merciful release."

Thoughts on euthanasia are usually grouped into the following categories:

1. *Eugenic mercy killing*—where the patient is a birth monster, hopelessly defective, incurably deranged, and so on.
2. *Active medical euthanasia*—where a drug is administered to hasten death.
3. *Passive euthanasia*—where a treatment is withheld even though it might technically prolong "life."

Passive euthanasia may consist of one of three forms:

1. Administering pain-killers in lethal dosages. (As the dosage of drugs must be constantly increased in order to have any effect, no doctor can be criticized if his patient's constitution cannot bear the increased dosage.)
2. *Stopping* treatment which is prolonging the patient's dying (i.e., turning off respirators, "pulling the plug").
3. Withholding treatment altogether.

There is also a distinction between *voluntary* and *involuntary* euthanasia. The first refers to those cases in which an adult wishes to have his life ended in order to save himself suffering. Within this category there are some other distinctions, but they have one common factor: *the person is asking to die.* Thus, voluntary euthanasia is actually a form of suicide that requires the assistance of others.

In England, as we have said, suicide is legal. Suppose, then, that an Englishman in a London hospital decides to pull the intravenous feeding tubes out of his arm. The hospital staff catch him at it and put the tubes back in. Could he then sue the hospital for conspiring to deprive him of his legal rights? Probably.

No doubt the situation would be even clearer in the United States, where there is an official written constitution. Supposing that the United States also allowed that suicide is legal. Promptly the American Civil Liberties Union would take up such a case as described above, for the patient's civil rights were clearly being interfered with. In no time at all a hospital might find itself thinking twice before pumping the sleeping pills out of some aging film star's stomach. Was she trying to commit suicide? Might she sue? No hospital could afford to take the chance.

*Involuntary* euthanasia involves killing someone without his permission for reasons which those who commit the killing feel are merciful. This category covers a wide spectrum: the murder of deformed babies or incurably sick children, stopping the heart-lung machine on a patient whose brain has died, increasing the drug dosage to ease, and shorten, the lives of dying patients, and even Nazi Germany's slaughter of innocents.

The medical profession does, of course, practice euthanasia —however you choose to define it—quite widely at its own discretion, but without calling public attention to the matter. Most likely doctors don't regard it as a controversial part of their work since it is so common. Articles have appeared in popular magazines where the doctor says, in effect: "She asked that she go to sleep and not wake up. She went to sleep and did not wake up." A few doctors would like to see euthanasia legalized in order to protect themselves, but by and large the medical profession bridles at the suggestion of interference with its traditional prerogatives.

It is interesting that the decision to terminate life by withholding some vital substance (artificially administered) or by discontinuing some artificially performed vital function is typically made with great secrecy and discretion. The average doctor would certainly not admit such things go on to the average newspaper reporter. The decision may be made by the physician without consultation with the patient's family. Certainly it is usually made without consulting a clergyman or lawyer. In a survey reported in the *Archives of Internal Medicine* for August, 1969, it was found that 87 percent of all American doctors were in favor of "passive" euthanasia, and that 80 percent had practiced it at some time or another. Even 81 percent of those *opposed* to euthanasia were in favor of "letting the patient go" when it seemed reasonable. According to an English poll, 76 percent of English doctors admitted helping their patients "over the edge": "In order to save them unnecessary suffering even if that involves some curtailment of life. . . ."

Generally, medical opinion on euthanasia is divided into three wide categories. First, there are those opposed to any deliberate shortening of life whatever. This group includes most Roman Catholic physicians, who do, however, on the advice of Pope Pius XII, among others, provide enough pain-killing drugs whose side effect is to shorten the life of the patient. The second group supports the belief that euthanasia is best left to the doctor's discretion. The majority of doctors probably fall into this category. Indeed, one of the rare medical textbooks which even deigns to discuss the subject, Davidson's *Medical Ethics* (1962), actually advocates killing the dying patient in special circumstances, and suggests suitable poisons. No mention is made of the patient's permission. The third group, and not the quietest by any means, is that small group of doctors who would like to see the law changed to permit voluntary euthanasia. Dr. Charlotte Gilman, when dying of cancer, wrote: "The time is approaching when we shall consider it abhorrent to our civilization to allow a human being to lie in prolonged agony which we should mercifully end in any other creature."

It is not surprising that doctors are forced to act in secrecy, or that some refuse to act at all. Although it is not very likely, given prevailing public opinion, that any doctor would go to prison for aiding the release of a hopelessly ill and pain-racked patient, some risk remains. A little extra morphine has for years been the physician's silent answer to the illegality of euthanasia. Society seems prepared to let the medical profession carry the burden of responsibility without real legal protection.

Do the doctors complain about this? On the contrary, they appear to prefer the laissez-faire policy. But in this situation the sufferer in every sense is the patient, dependent on the views, conscience, or even courage of his own doctor. And it must be recognized that a small minority of doctors still rigidly interpret their medical duty as the preservation of "life" at all costs.

Not long ago, Sir George Pickering, Regius Professor of Medicine at Oxford University, addressed himself to the question: "Should one keep certain very sick patients alive indefinitely?":

> A distinguished scientist whom I knew very well had a series of strokes. He couldn't walk, he couldn't talk, he was bedridden, he had to be fed, and he was incontinent both in the urine and feces; and he was looked after by his devoted wife, who was unable to go out of the house the last year of his life. The last time I went to see him he was breathing at 40 [breaths] per minute and I knew that he had bronchial pneumonia. Should I have informed his physician so that he could give him antibiotics? . . . What I did was to say nothing, and four days later that man died. And that I think was right, because this was ruining a devoted woman's life.

Should doctors and nurses be licensed to kill? Most people would say "No!" But that is what they do, every day, through a consciously chosen neglect. One doctor has said: "I have no sympathy with the man who would shorten the death agony of a dog but prolong that of a human being. . . ." And this physician once advised a class of medical students: "I hold it to be your duty to smooth as much as possible the pathway to the grave even if life is somewhat shortened. Nor is it necessary to talk it over with friends and relatives nor need you expect them to formally countenance either neglect or expedition. Let that be your affair, settled with your own conscience."

Perhaps more than we know, euthanasia is today largely an academic question. At a recent meeting of physicians in New York City the chairman requested a show of hands of those physicians who had never administered euthanasia. Not one hand was raised.

The positions of the religions are far more permissive on euthanasia than is popularly supposed. One group that one might expect to be most opposed to any hastening of death, namely, Orthodox Jews, is not in principle opposed. Rabbi Imanuel Jakobovits, writing in his book, *Jewish Medical Ethics* (1959), which is usually accepted as a standard for the Orthodox view, assents to "the legality of expediting the death of an incurable patient in acute agony by withholding from him such medicaments as sustain his continued life by unnatural means."

The Roman Catholic view is better known. Pope Pius XII, in a series of addresses in the 1950s, gave a clear statement to the Catholic view on many questions of medical ethics. He pointed out that there was no absolute obligation for the physician to employ extraordinary means to preserve life. Extraordinary means were defined as those that cannot be used or obtained without undue expense, pain, or other inconvenience, and that offer no reasonable hope or benefit. Further, Pope Pius defended the administration of a pain-killer to relieve pain in the knowledge that it might, as a secondary result, end the patient's life, thus falling back on the ancient principle of the rule of double effect.

There is probably a greater willingness in religious circles than in almost any other area to look upon the aims of euthanasia favorably. I know of no moral grounds in any faith that would argue against stopping treatment, or indeed not starting treatment, of a patient facing a miserable death if that treatment merely served biological prolongation.

The basis of Christian opposition to euthanasia is not that life has paramount value, but rather that it is up to God to dispose of it. But how, then, are we to account for the myriad chaplains accompanying all Christian armies, encouraging them to slaughter each other, always, on either side, "in the name of God"?

In the United States, polls on euthanasia usually indicate that opinion is against it. In England, however, the majority is usually in favor. In 1939 it was found that 46 percent of Americans and 60 percent of the British favored some sort of legal euthanasia. A poll by England's *Public Opinion Quarterly* in 1950 revealed that on the question of whether to end the life of a person with an incurable illness, opinion was divided about evenly, with a significantly larger number of women opposed. There was also a significantly larger number opposed among those over fifty. The euthanasiasts are fond of pointing out that this survey mentioned only incurability, which is surely less serious than excruciating pain or loss of functionality. Recent polls have also established that 75 percent of all general practitioners in England favor euthanasia laws.

To most of us, administering euthanasia to the senile seems unthinkable, but it should be considered in the context of a community that can no longer adequately nurse its sick, where the long-term usage of hospital beds by the hopelessly ill aged means the denial of those beds and nursing services to younger sick people with a good chance of recovery. We can no longer avoid the issue of medicated survival which, as currently practiced, surely may be one of the cruelest hazards for aging people. As Dr. Kenneth Vickery puts it: "The Bible clearly indicates that those who survive to fourscore years may pay dearly for their extra time in suffering and sorrow."

Many people believe that the Ten Commandments proscribe killing. This is a common misconception. Actually, in the correct translation, the Sixth Commandment reads: "Thou shalt do no murder." And murder is defined as malicious killing. It's a rare doctor who kills out of maliciousness.

Still more confusing is the fact that the various euthanasia societies and their opposing "human rights" groups in the United States and England often appear to be working at cross-purposes. For example, here is a statement from one of these groups—can you guess which?

> . . . Just how long should an unconscious patient be *artificially* kept alive when there is no reasonable hope of recovery . . . is a purely technical question as to the stage at which hope must be given up. A very hard decision, but

not different in principle from many that have been made before when rescue operations have had to be abandoned for trapped miners or vessels lost at sea. Deliberate killing is not involved.

By the euthanasiasts? No. From their opponents, specifically Britain's Human Rights Society. One begins to suspect that the two groups are really in agreement, except that the anti-euthanasiasts prefer the status quo—that is, with doctors secretly making all the decisions in these areas in an extra-legal, ad lib fashion. Even a leading spokesman for the anti-euthanasia forces in England can say:

> A doctor . . . is under a duty to preserve life. . . . That does not mean that there is a duty to prolong life at any cost. That would neither be good morality nor good medicine. Lord Horder [the chief opponent of the 1936 euthanasia bill] . . . once said that the good doctor will know how to distinguish between prolonging life and prolonging the act of dying.

In brief, the human rightists are not opposed to passive euthanasia for those beyond the pale.

The leading argument of the voluntary euthanasiasts for legalization is that it would allow that small proportion of individuals who are dying in great suffering to ease their deaths. According to Professor J. M. Hinton in his widely quoted book *Dying*:

> Whenever this problem is considered there always lingers in the mind the thought that euthanasia should so rarely be necessary. The suffering during fatal illness ought to be

better relieved. But while the dying do sometimes experience anguish, even if in theory it could have been alleviated, the fact that euthanasia could have curtailed much distress for some people cannot be entirely dismissed. As long as one can truly say that for the patient merciful death has been too long in coming, there is some justification for euthanasia.

Or, as the Reverend A. B. Downing puts it in his excellent *Euthanasia and the Right to Death*:

By the bed of an actual sufferer the proportions of the problem are seen quite differently. It becomes no longer a question of the sanctity of "life" and the need to prolong a suffering existence just as long as it is technically possible, but a case in which the compelling demands of compassion and dignity combine to impose a quick and merciful death as the only *natural* solution.

And Eliot Slater, in *Man, Mind and Heredity*, writes:

[it is argued that] even if the most energetic treatment is only likely to secure a few more days of life, it should not be spared. Now, of course, there is no logical limit to this line of argument. If the duty of the medical man is to be assessed in this way, then he must disturb the dying man to provide him with a few more hours, indeed a few more minutes or even moments; and the last injection of coramine will take precedence over the wish of the wife to say farewell.

One woman confined to a wheelchair for thirteen years with rheumatoid arthritis has explained her position on voluntary euthanasia:

I cannot wash, dress or get in or out of bed. Drugs have ruined my eyesight, depriving me of the pleasure of reading and television, and I am too crippled to even work a gramaphone. I am physically dependent on another invalid who might have to give up at any time. The spectre of *complete* helplessness haunts me, and this anguish could be banished if lawful euthanasia were possible. I could live much more happily if I knew that I could ask my doctor to end my miseries when they became intolerable.

Contrary to the conventional wisdom, suffering is anything but ennobling. The hard truth is that it is a destructive force that usually reduces both body and spirit to something less than human. Dr. Charlotte Gilman, herself dying horribly of cancer, wrote before taking her own life: "When all usefulness is over, when one is assured of an imminent and unavoidable death, it is the simplest of human rights to choose a quick and easy death in place of a slow and horrible one. I have preferred chloroform to cancer."

Dr. Gilman, of course, had the medical means at hand, but for most of those ill enough to want it, suicide is not always easy. A Vietnam War veteran, stricken by a crippling progressive disease and able to move only the fingers of one hand, managed somehow to get his head inside a plastic bag in a desperate effort to escape the dying his doctors had prescribed for him. He was found and revived to face the harsh fact that unless he could get some assistance from somewhere, he could never succeed on his own. A proud man, used to command, he now dreads the daily humiliations of his utter dependence, and above all dreads the inevitable daily progression of his disease as it finally clouds and deranges his formerly keen mind

On the other hand, even a former officer of the Euthanasia Society of America has said: "Very few incurables have or express the wish to die. However great their physical suffering may be, the will to live, the desire for life, is such an overwhelming force that pain and suffering become bearable. . . ." And diagnosis of what is "curable" and what is not may be quite fallible. Dr. Benjamin Miller was left to die as a "hopeless" tuberculosis victim, only to discover that he was in actuality suffering from a rare disease with similar symptoms that rarely kills. A useful illustration of the fallibility of diagnosis has been presented by Miller in this recollection of the last diagnostic clinic of the brilliant Dr. Richard Cabot on the occasion of his official retirement:

> He was given the case records of two patients and asked to diagnose their illnesses. . . . The patients had died and only the hospital pathologist knew the exact diagnosis beyond doubt. . . . Dr. Cabot, usually very accurate in his diagnosis, that day missed both. . . . The chief pathologist who had selected the cases was a wise person. He had purposely chosen two of the most deceptive to remind the medical students and young physicians that even at the end of a long and rich experience one of the greatest diagnosticians of our time was still not infallible.

Consider the case of a thirty-eight-year-old woman who was brought into a hospital in England after a frightful automobile accident. She was deeply unconscious and neurological study determined the prognosis to be zero. Consequently the doctors did not set the fractures in her legs, believing that she would die shortly. Miraculously, the woman began to recover, and it was too late to set her fractures. For how much should she sue the hospital?

An American doctor also reminds us: ". . . I have personally seen persons abandoned by one doctor for supposedly incurable cancer, relieved and sometimes cured by others more courageous, so this is rather dangerous ice to get on."

K. S. Jones in the *Medical Journal of Australia* explains how easy it is to make an error in judgment:

> I well remember on one occasion my own embarrassment as a very new casualty surgeon at the Royal Prince Alfred Hospital. The ambulance attendants rushed in with a large, pale man lying on a stretcher and called "Quick doctor!" I . . . found an inert body with a bullet hole over the line of the abdominal aorta. The pulses were absent and the respiration had ceased, so I pronounced life to be extinct. No sooner had I done so than the patient took a deep breath! I hastily reversed my edict, but the poor chap then refused permanently to give any sign of life.

Dr. Lawrence A. Kohn has reported some of "my many mistakes" in the *Medical Times*:

> . . . in a woman of forty-five, the diagnosis of sclerderma was made, clinically and by biopsy in 1944. The sections were recently reviewed and the diagnosis was correct, but the multiple lesions receded and the woman is well. . . .
>
> A seventy-year-old lawyer was admitted to the hospital comatose, paralyzed on one side. In the next twenty-four

hours, he developed high fever, auricular fibrillation and pulmonary oedema. The spinal fluid was grossly bloody. I gave the family a verdict of "no hope." He recovered and practiced at the bar with minimal residue damage for two years.

There are also so-called miraculous recoveries, admittedly very rare. People have been apparently dead up to nine hours only to spontaneously recover. An equally minute number of incurables may be suddenly saved by the discovery of some new cure. For example, a patient suffering from pemphigus, a skin disease, was about to die when a new penicillin was flown in from another city. He disappointed priest and family by recovering! How many apparent candidates for euthanasia were rescued by the introduction of insulin, malaria pills, the new successful treatments for liver ailments, X-rays, and radium? In 1922, a man suffering from diabetes was an incurable. In 1923, he could be saved by insulin.

An old doctor who made me promise him anonymity provides the following illustration of why he is to this day somewhat doubtful about euthanasia:

It was the notice of his death in the daily paper one day that brought it all back to me. The notice was one of the usual brief, bald statements of obituary; his age was eighty-one years. He was an old man, and he had outlived those of his friends that mattered. He had achieved no eminence, nor had he occupied any sort of public position. He was a poor farmer, the owner of a poor farm in one of the poor parts of the country. And when I had last known him he had been a much younger man—in his middle thirties.

## THE GODS OF LIFE

He came under my care about forty-seven years ago, when I was working in a hospital where he had been admitted. He had paid many visits to the hospital; each time it was the same story. He came in tired, yellow, weak, and breathless. Rest in bed, good food, and a transfusion of blood, and he would go home temporarily improved. The intervals between visits, however, were getting shorter, the transfusions more frequent, and the effect more transient. We usually got a friend to volunteer to give his blood and at the beginning we had almost too many offers, but after a time the friends seemed to disappear—the novelty wore off and nothing seemed to be given in return. It is hard to keep one's sympathy always green.

This next visit to the hospital was only twelve days after his previous one. He was spending almost as much time with us as at home, and the precious blood we were giving him seemed to be wasted. It could not go on like this. Things came to a head one Sunday afternoon when I was able to discuss the situation with his wife. I tried to be as kind as I could in explaining the bad news—yes, he was going to die, the case was hopeless; he was no longer making his own fresh blood and was only being kept alive by the blood of others. This state of affairs was impossible. Yes, we would help any way we could, but since she had to come such a long way from the country to visit, perhaps it were best if he died in his own home. It would certainly be easier to move him at this stage than any later one.

And so the incident was finished, and we made arrangements to send him home, there gradually to sink into his final decline. I dreaded those few hopeless weeks that his wife, some years his senior, would have to spend watching him lose his battle for life. The thought was in my head: "Why not help to speed his end and save them both that agonizing struggle?"

But then the latest medical journal arrived. It contained the usual mixed budget of views and information; but in one corner I noticed something on the treatment of anemia with liver . . . raw liver in large quantities and entirely uncooked. It seemed absurd that liver should differ from meat in general; it probably was absurd. Very likely the cases quoted had not been the real thing and certainly they could not have been as murderous as what was overtaking my patient.

But on the other hand, my patient was dying . . . so what did it matter if the treatment was worthless or not? No doubt I would have prescribed raw mud if I had read anything good about it.

On Monday he started. The usual opposition from the kitchen over special dieting, and from the nurses, was overcome. (Remember, this was 1923—the doctor did not have the dictatorial power he has today in hospitals.) He took his dose daily like a man; pounded, grated, squeezed, mixed, always horrible looking for any civilized man, and always raw. Even the heavy seasoning we put into it would not have deceived me. Then Friday came and he was somewhat better. . . .

His pulse was now slower, his cheeks not so yellow. The days went by. The improvement continued, the atmosphere changed, and even the nurses became convinced that something strange was happening. His wife came to bring him home to die and was astonished at our decision that he remain in the hospital.

The following weeks bore us out. Six weeks later—he was by then up daily and walking around the ward—he was able to leave the hospital under his own power. It was in a way sad to see him go. He was in some sense our creation, our success, and yet six weeks before I would have written his death certificate or even given him something to shorten his time.

Thus, when people talk of euthanasia, I always remember my young man with the anemia, and I wonder what will be in tomorrow's medical journal. We never saw him again —that was a good sign—but we would have liked to shake his hand. Today his wife is long dead. So you can understand how his obituary called up a vivid memory, and you will understand why I feel that I have lost a friend.

# The Living Will:
## One Legal Aspect

The prospect of legalizing the right to a merciful death raises many important moral, social, medical, and legal questions. One suggestion that is currently gaining considerable acceptance is that people be permitted, under the law, to make out wills authorizing the practice of euthanasia on their persons in the event that they are seriously and irreversibly incapacitated or otherwise reduced to a nonfunctioning state.

One of the leading crusaders on the American scene for the "living will" is attorney Luis Kutner. Mr. Kutner, a nominee twice for the Nobel Prize for Peace (1962 and 1972), is also the originator of the World Habeas Corpus concept, which opposes the arbitrary detention of persons all over the world. He is currently at work on a book dealing with World Habeas Corpus—*The Human Right to Individual Freedom*—with Arthur J. Goldberg, former Supreme Court Justice and Ambassador to the United Nations.

It is a privilege to reprint here, with permission, a portion excerpted from one of Mr. Kutner's recent articles on the "living will" originally published in the *Indiana Law Journal*.

## THE LIVING WILL

The law provides that a patient may not be subjected to treatment without his consent. But when he is in a condition in which his consent cannot be expressed, the physician must assume that the patient wishes to be treated to preserve his life. His failure to act fully to keep the patient alive in a particular instance may lead to liability for negligence. But it may well be that a patient does not desire to be kept in a state of indefinite vegetated animation. How then can the individual patient retain the right of privacy over his body— the right to determine whether he should be permitted to die, to permit his body to be given to the undertaker?

The law clearly prohibits mercy killing, even if undertaken at the patient's request. Thus, the patient cannot request another to end his life. Such an action would subject the actor to prosecution for murder. But an individual does have the right to refuse to permit a doctor to treat him, even if such treatment would prolong his life. If a doctor should act contrary to his wishes, he would be subject to liability.

Where a patient undergoes surgery or other radical treatment, the surgeon or the hospital will require him to sign a legal statement indicating his consent to the treatment. The patient, however, while still retaining his mental faculties and the ability to convey his thoughts, could append to such a document a clause providing that, if his condition becomes incurable and his bodily state vegetative with no possibility that he could recover his complete faculties, his consent to further treatment would be terminated. The physician would then be precluded from prescribing further surgery, radiation, drugs or the running of resuscitating and other machinery, and the patient would be permitted to die by virtue of the physician's inaction.

The patient may not have had, however, the opportunity to give his consent at any point before treatment. He may have become the victim of a sudden accident or a stroke or coronary. Therefore, the suggested solution is that the individual, while fully in control of his faculties and his ability to express himself, indicate to what extent he would consent to treatment. The document indicating such consent may be referred to as "a *living will*," "a declaration determining the termination of life," "testament permitting death," "declaration for bodily autonomy," "declaration for ending treatment," "body trust," or other similar reference.

The document would provide that if the individual's bodily

state becomes completely vegetative and it is certain that he cannot regain his mental and physical capacities, medical treatment shall cease. A Jehovah's Witness whose religious principles are opposed to blood transfusions could so provide in such a document. A Christian Scientist could, by virtue of such a document, indicate that he does not wish any medical treatment.

The document would be notarized and attested to by at least two witnesses who would affirm that the maker was of sound mind and acted of his own free will. The individual could carry the document on his person at all times, while his wife, his personal physician, a lawyer or confidant would have the original copy.

Each individual case would be referred to a hospital committee, board or a committee of physicians. A precedent for the functioning of such committees or boards already exists in many hospitals for determining whether an abortion is medically necessary. The committee or board would consider the circumstances under which the document was made in determining the patient's intent and also make a determination as to whether the condition of the patient has indeed reached the point where he would no longer want any treatment.

The individual could at any time, before reaching the comatose state, revoke the document. Personal possession of the document would create a strong presumption that he regards it as still binding. Statements and actions subsequent to the writing of the document may indicate a contrary intent. If the physicians find that some doubt exists as to the patient's intent, they would give treatment pending the resolution of the matter. The document, if carried on the patient's person, should indicate what persons should be contacted if he reaches a comatose state. The physician would consult with them in making a determination.

A *living will* could only be made by a person who is capable of giving his consent to treatment. A person who is a minor, institutionalized, or adjudged incompetent could not make such a declaration. A guardian should not be permitted to make such a declaration on behalf of his ward nor a parent on behalf of his child. If an individual makes a *living will* and is subsequently adjudged incompetent, the *will* would be deemed to be revoked. However, this revocation would not apply where the state of incompetency resulted from the medical condition which was contemplated in making the declaration.

The *living will* is analogous to a revocable or conditional trust with the patient's body as the *res*, the patient as the beneficiary and grantor, and the doctor and hospital as the trustees. The doctor is given authority to act as the trustee of the patient's body by virtue of the patient's consent to treatment. He is obligated to exercise due care and is subject to liability for negligence. The patient is free at any time to revoke the trust. From another perspective, the patient in giving consent to treatment is limiting the authority the doctor and other medical persons may exercise over his body. The patient has the ultimate right to decide what is to be done with him and may not irrevocably confer authority on somebody else. The patient may not be compelled to undergo treatment contrary to his *will*. He should not be compelled to take certain drugs, receive inoculations or therapy or undergo surgery without his express assent. At any point he may stop treatment or he may change physicians.

One problem to be encountered by the *living will* concept is mental illness. An individual who becomes mentally ill has the same rights as any other patient. He may, by the *living will,* anticipate mental illness and limit his consent to treatment accordingly. If in the course of his mental illness he enters an incurable comatose state, treatment may cease. The problem, however, is that, on becoming mentally ill, the court may find him incompetent and appoint a guardian.

Could or should the guardian revoke the *living will* or is it deemed to have become revoked? Here the approach of the trust concept is suggested. The trust relationship between the doctor and the patient was created by the *living will* with the patient as grantor. It was the patient's intent, in creating the trust and drawing the trust document—the *living will*—to cover contingencies wherein he would be incapable of granting or withholding assent to treatment. Incompetency because of mental illness is precisely such a situation. Therefore, the *living will* remains in effect. The guardian may not nullify it. However, when the patient is mentally ill, he may still have instances when his mind is lucid. During such instances he may indicate to his guardian that he wishes the *will* revoked and the guardian could then act accordingly. He might also indicate this intent to the physician who would so inform the guardian and have the *will* revoked.

The *living will* may be used within another context affecting a mentally ill patient. In agreeing to be committed for treatment to a hospital, he could condition the kind of treatment to be given to him. By voluntarily committing himself he does not automatically confer upon the doctor the right to perform a lobotomy, insulin or electric shock therapy, to deny him the right to choose another doctor, to deny him the right to receive visitors or to enjoy other rights. The *living will* could provide that he be released from the hospital if he fails to receive any treatment or does not respond to therapy. If he is confined against his will, the *living will* could be used as a basis for invoking a writ of habeas corpus to effectuate his release.

The *living will* is limited in its initial creation to adult patients who are capable of exercising their will. It applies to those patients who have the right to decide whether they may receive treatment. It does not apply to a parent acting on behalf of his child. Thus, while an adult patient may refuse to undergo an operation or receive a blood transfusion which will save his life, a parent may not deprive a child of such treatment. Though the state recognizes the rights of parents in relation to their children, it acts *in loco parentis* to protect the rights of the children. But the state may not interfere to infringe upon the rights of a mature individual as to the disposition of his body; the law is required to protect the autonomy of the patient.

However, while a patient may determine the type of medical treatment he may receive, he may not use the *living will* as a means for directing a doctor or another individual to *act* affirmatively to terminate his life. He may not authorize the commission of euthanasia. The Law of Trusts recognizes that certain types of trusts for certain designated purposes may be contrary to public policy. Similarly, a *living will* authorizing

THE GODS OF LIFE

mercy killing is contrary to public policy. In this instance, public policy considerations outweigh the apparent rights of the patient. The basic function of the law is to protect human life. Because of the possibility that, if mercy killing be permitted without judicial controls, an individual would be killed contrary to his will and the law now extant cannot permit legalized euthanasia. The right to life is basic and the possibility of some persons being murdered regardless of their *will* means that euthanasia may not be condoned. Therefore, as of now, a doctor cannot be directed to act affirmatively to terminate a patient's life. He may, however, be directed and exculpated to act passively by inaction. However, the patient's *living will* adjudicated by a court and buttressed by medical and lay testimony and evidence, can create the affirmative inaction termination of a patient's life. This can be resorted to in instances where the hospital board on euthanasia may decline to assume the responsibility.

# Hope for the
# Future

PART IV

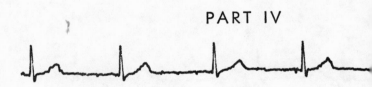

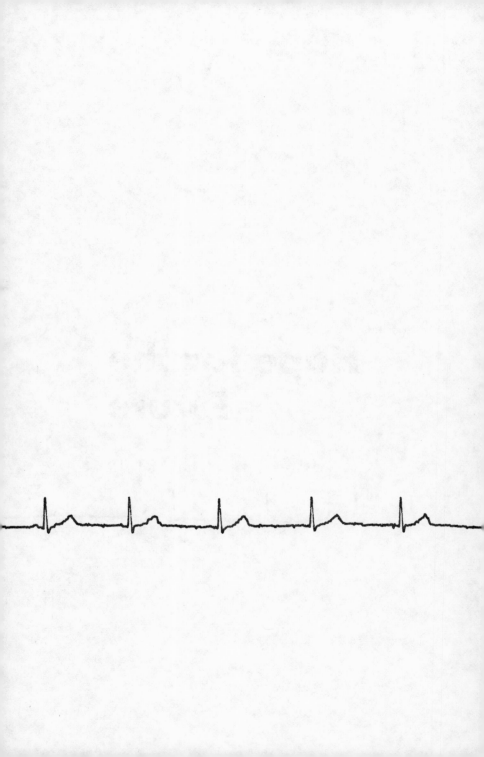

# Cadaver Man:
## The Great Transplant Hoax

*It's cheaper to make new models.*

—Alexandrei Breznhev, Chairman of
the Medical Councils, Soviet Union

## THE GODS OF LIFE

The surgical techniques are now available for virtually any organ's transplant. But the organs we will most likely see transplanted are the liver, kidney, heart, and lung.

Earlier in this century Charles C. Guthrie was acknowledged as the first doctor to graft a second head onto a dog and to transfer the lung and heart of a kitten into the neck of a cat. The Russians, out of their usual scientific jealousy, naturally went ahead in the thirties and grafted a second head onto one of *their* dogs. Both heads salivated, rolled their eyes, and performed other important functions that contributed a lot to medical science. The returns are not yet all in on the value of these operations, though such progress may someday give greater meaning to that ancient expression, "Two heads are better than one."

A Belgian surgeon has perfected the art of right-lung transplant, and this operation is now being tried in the United States. Recipients of lung transplants have survived briefly, for just weeks. Almost a hundred liver transplants have been done, and a few of the recipients have lived almost a year. Elsewhere, a new pancreas has been stitched into a patient's neck. In the future one may be able to purchase new organs in some kind of medical supermarket. And someday perhaps the government will record our organs on IBM cards the way it now records blood types and fingerprints. A man's body, however he dies, may automatically go into the national organ bank.

The best known transplant operation, of course, is of the heart. It has become something of a cliché in this age of medical marvels to say that it's easier to find a doctor to transplant a heart than to find one who will treat a sore throat.

Actually, Christiaan Barnard wasn't there first. According to Ilza Veith, a medical historian of the University of California, the first heart was transplanted into General Kuan Kung in the third century A.D. in China. (This was probably the first case on record of a soldier losing his heart to his general.) Dr. Barnard did launch a trend on December 3, 1967, however, when he successfully transplanted the heart of a dead girl into the chest of a dying man. The heart transplant boom had begun and suddenly the number of heart transplants performed around the world increased dramatically. Five transplants took place between December 3 and January 9, 1968. By the end of 1968 there had been ninety-seven transplants, all well publicized. Without doubt the heart transplant was one of the miracles of twentieth-century medicine.

Then the bubble burst. By August, 1969, the number of heart transplants performed in the world had dropped to forty-five in a year, and only twenty-two have been done since then. Some doctors say there's an unofficial moratorium on heart transplants.

In actuality, the box score for heart transplants is not very good—but who counts? All the public hears about is the successful transplant. Usually little is said when the patient dies inauspiciously several weeks later. *Only 3 percent of the recipients live more than 6 months.* Only 13 percent live more than an hour. By any standard the operation has not been very successful.

**151**

## THE GODS OF LIFE

A gauge of the true judgment of experts on the reliability of the transplant emerged from a 1968 poll of cardiologists taken by the Marion Laboratories of Kansas City, Missouri: more than half the specialists claimed that they would not agree to heart transplant for themselves "even if they had advanced heart disease with a poor prognosis." Very enlightening.

The least controversial and most successful aspect of heart transplant is the surgical technique. Basically a cutting and stitching procedure, it involves removing the heart of a person who has just died and using it to replace a diseased heart. The difficulties lie in matching the donor's blood to the recipient's, obtaining a heart that is close to the recipient's in size, getting the newly transplanted organ to beat properly, and making sure the patient's body does not reject the foreign tissue. Most heart specialists point to the rejection phenomenon as the major cause of the slowdown in heart transplants. They also say it accounts for the low survival rate. Dr. Barnard acknowledged the problem at the start when he told the press that sooner or later rejection would necessitate a second heart transplant for even the most successful recipients.

What happens is that the body's immunological system (a marshalling of white blood cells) destroys any foreign tissue—whether a splinter, a pneumonia germ, or a transplanted heart. The degree of tissue compatibility is a factor here, because drugs can control rejection when the donor is a relative. Of course, most heart transplants rely on nonrelative sources, and doctors cannot give immuno-suppressive drugs in high enough dosages to prevent rejection without simultane-

**152**

ously endangering the patient's life. Since these powerful drugs reduce the body's ability to defend against infections, potentially the simplest germ can kill the recovering heart transplant patient.

A medical research team at the University of Chicago Billings Memorial Hospital is experimenting with a technique to specifically suppress the body's immune mechanism to an organ transplant. A surgeon there says: "Our angle is to try and play a trick on the patient's immunological system. Most of the drugs that prevent rejection are nonspecific. We want to specifically impair the recipient's ability to react to the determinants in the donor organ." However, the antirejection technique is still in the animal experimentation stage. The researchers say that the concept is relatively simple, but there are problems in determining working doses, antibodies, and tissue extracts that can be used to get the patient "turned off" ahead of time. Synthetic grafts often work when human ones won't, simply because they contain no organic matter. Millions of years of evolution have scarcely equipped the white blood cells to identify plastic. The blood will accept Dacron, and form fibers around it very quickly so that the entire foreign part becomes in a sense a dressmaker's dummy upon which to hang the body's cells.

It is hard to realize that heart transplant has been going on only for several years. In 1967 doctors in New York and Palo Alto were ready to transplant. But Dr. Norman Shumway had no donor, Dr. Kantrowitz wasn't quite *that* ready, and Walter DeBakey was still researching the matter. Then the world heard about Dr. Christiaan Barnard and a plumber named Louis Washkansky.

Barnard transplanted. The world watched Washkansky "with obscenely bated breath." As soon as Washkansky came out of ether, microphones were thrust at his lips and TV carried his message around the world via satellite.

"Say it again, Lou," demanded the reporter.

"The doctor," gasped the plumber who would live to be enshrined in the encyclopedias of forty-eight nations, "the doctor is the man with the golden hands. . . ."

Two days later Washkansky died.

Barnard's next candidate, a Capetown dentist named Dr. Blaiberg, was luckier. While Blaiberg lived, the world waited anxiously upon his daily medical report. He sent out autographed pictures of himself to his public, and spoke of himself as a celebrity. Although it took fifty years for Dr. Blaiberg's first heart to become so clogged with fats and cholesterol that it failed, it took less than two for his second heart to become similarly diseased. And that second heart had come from the chest of a healthy twenty-four-year-old. The message is ironic: the man who needs a transplant most is probably the last person in the world who should have one.

The blood vessels of Blaiberg's second heart were more heavily choked with fats than any others South African pathologist Dr. J. G. Thomson had seen in forty years of autopsies. It was as if Blaiberg's body had been hustling overtime to bring the second heart to the level of his first. The sudden shift from a healthy body into Blaiberg's atherosclerotic one was just too much for the heart. The fatty deposits settled everywhere, rather than just in the usual few places. By the time he expired, Blaiberg's two-year-old heart (twenty-six years old, really) was in worse condition than his fifty-eight-year-old one had been. The sole reason Blaiberg survived so long was that his new blood vessels clogged with singular uniformity instead of developing concentrated weak spots of the sort that usually cause sudden heart attacks. Thus, his blood vessels were too thickly armored with fat to suddenly "blow out." But they were so narrow that his heart had to strain terribly to force the blood through. Ironically, the second heart failed merely because it was so young and healthy it had not had the time to slowly build up its defenses to fat-clogging.

Philip Blaiberg lived almost twenty months with his transplanted heart, setting a record. Although he was depicted all along as hale and hearty as a Rotarian greeter, a recent book by his widow reveals that actually he was miserably uncomfortable, if not downright ill, during most of his life with his new heart. Since Blaiberg's death, Louis B. Russell, Jr., a Negro schoolteacher from Indianapolis, has surpassed his record for longevity. Russell had four crises resulting from his body's "rejection" of the strange heart, but immuno-suppressive drugs brought him around in time. Russell's case is also unique in that he has continued to work hard teaching carpentry at an industrial arts school. In short, unlike the other transplant recipients, he does manual work, and therein may lie the difference.

Rejection isn't the only hazard in heart transplant. Autopsy studies of patients who lived more than a few weeks with borrowed hearts showed a rapid buildup of fibrous tissue in the arteries of the heart. This swift growth of tissue may almost completely block the flow of blood to the heart. This finding led Montreal surgeons to halt transplant operations last year. They believe the thickening is part of the rejection process and are awaiting more research before they resume transplants.

In the meantime, noisy conflict has built up over the question of when an individual can be considered dead "enough" to have his heart donated to the body of another person. Obviously, if the transplant surgeon must wait until the heart is definitively "dead," this seriously curtails the possibility that the donated heart will be viable in a new body. On the other hand, there is something obscene about surgeons hovering like vultures over someone who is about to "go under" so that they can rip out his still-beating heart.

The publicity about heart transplants has obscured other developments. For example, *either human or animal bone* can be used to link the ends of a fractured bone and support it while it regrows. The transplanted bone must also bridge the gap between the fractured ends, in order to prevent scars from developing which might block the regrowing bone. White blood cells cannot enter bone, so rejection is no problem, and the grafted bone will gradually be absorbed and disposed of naturally by the bone cells.

*Heart valves* as well lack blood vessels, and thus can be replaced by valves from corpses. Valves from pigs have also worked well, as the pig's heart is most similar to our own.

Many people feel that pigs' hearts may be the wave of the future. (We do not have the pigs' opinion on this.)

*Arteries* can be replaced from the body itself, as a "spare" artery can be made from vein. When veins are removed, a new channel is automatically created in their place by the circulatory system, and the removed vein can then be stitched onto an artery by simple surgery.

Transplanting the *cornea* from the eye of a dead donor is common, and thousands of people yearly will their eyes to "eye banks." Success with eye transplants is due largely to the absence of a direct blood supply to the cornea.

The *kidney* is somewhat outside the body's complex immunity system, which may explain why kidney transplants have worked so well. The problem of rejection has been mitigated by tissue typing, a system of locating the elements in tissue cells that can avoid rejection. Complexities aside, the results of this system have been excellent. Consequently, with related donors in cases of kidney transplant, 90 percent today live more than a year, and with unrelated donors success has increased to 79 percent.

Because they come in pairs, kidneys are good candidates for transplant, since a person can live with just one. Initially only kidney transplants between identical twins worked, but new white cell suppressants have made kidney transplant relatively routine.

Doctors have also opened up the possibility of using kidneys from corpses, though they face a lot of obstacles with this method. First they must sustain the heart and lungs of the "corpse" so that the kidney doesn't deteriorate; then they must get the approval of next-of-kin if the dead person has not given his consent previously; and finally the kidney must be transferred swiftly to the hospital where it will be transplanted. In the meantime, the patient needing the kidney must be prepared for the operation. Then, at the last possible moment, the diseased kidney is removed. With a live donor the tricky switch can be done in one operating room with two surgical teams working side by side.

*Liver* transplants are most unusual. Pigs' livers have kept a woman alive for eighteen days. They have been transplanted into people many times, but rejection usually occurs after only a few weeks. One way of trying to sidestep rejection is to utilize the new liver externally. Externally? Yes. The pig's liver is kept in a glass box and linked to the patient by tubes inserted into both an artery and a vein in the arm. Blood is circulated out through these tubes into a solution which prevents it from clotting, and then into the pig's liver, which carries out many of the normal functions the patient's own liver can no longer handle. Doctors hope that this "vacation" relief will give the old human liver some chance to recuperate and regenerate. Each pig's liver is used for several hours, then thrown away. During such an operation the patient typically regains power, even though previously he may have been in a coma and dying. However, if the patient's liver does not eventually regenerate, death is inevitable after several weeks.

All transplant operations involve a question of priorities. According to a distinguished English physician, money spent on one of Dr. Barnard's heart transplants could have been used to save the lives of two hundred undernourished African children. Heart transplants are now a matter of national prestige, "but," asks the English doctor, "is it justifiable to keep an operating theater on *heart* transplants if you have fifty, sixty, seventy, or more young men whose functional capacity is impaired by a hernia which could be cured in a matter of weeks or months?" In short, the breakthrough in heart transplant must be considered against the background of increasing tuberculosis and appalling malnutrition among South Africans. Dr. Blaiberg's operation must be seen in the social context of an area where 50 percent of all children die before the age of five.

An average of ten thousand Americans die yearly because there are not enough kidney machines or transplants. A heart transplant costs up to $75,000 and may require as many as twenty-five doctors. Who should pay for it? A kidney transplant could cost up to $22,000. For $1.5 billion we could save the twenty-five thousand or more kidney disease patients who will need transplants or dialysis in the next ten years. But for the same amount of money we could extend the routine health care that most of us take for granted to hundreds of thousands of poor people who desperately need it. *What should our priorities be?*

# A New You:
## Man or Robot?

*All flesh is as grass.*

—The New Covenant

Though organ transplants have received a great deal of publicity, the perfecting of artificial body parts may soon make transplanting a "dead" science. The cadaver-heart transplant will someday be to the artificial heart what the old icebox is to today's refrigerator. Many doctors think that eventually all of our parts will be replaceable.

Actually, medical technology is still at a primitive stage, although it is fast advancing. It is less than fifty years since Philip Drinker produced the first clumsy iron lung. Yet already people are wearing myoelectric hands that can pick up a dime and hand it to you without your noticing that the hand is artificial. We have kidney machines. In the next few years, we could be carrying silicone hearts or man-made livers and lungs. A bit later, but certainly, there will be electronic eyes. It is possible that such small items could be perfected and mass-produced at a low enough price to put them on the counter at Woolworth's. ("Oh, Harry, go down to the shopping center and pick me up a new eye, will you? This one got scratched yesterday.") Unquestionably the day is not too far off when people will have all of their organs replaced at age thirty with artificial ones, purely for convenience or custom. Just as today we continue to take smallpox shots even though there has been no smallpox in the Western Hemisphere for many decades. When that happens, will we be men, or will we be robots?

The *artificial kidney* was devised in 1944 by Dutch surgeon Willen Kolff. It was used at first only in sterile hospital rooms, then on general wards, and finally home use was made possible with the development of the Scribner shunt. This artificial diversion (two plastic tubes permanently implanted in an artery and vein in the forearm) can be connected to tubes leading to a filter unit. Blood from the patient flows past a membrane separating it from a special solution; the wastes in the blood cross the membrane into the fluid, but the rest of the blood cannot pass through.

In the human kidneys, each weighing roughly six ounces and measuring about four and one-half by two and one-half by one inches, wastes are filtered through two million microscopic units—a million to each kidney. The synthetic membrane in the artificial kidney must, therefore, be very fine. Made up of pores about eight-millionths of a millimeter in diameter, the membrane allows only water and molecular wastes to filter through; larger molecules of blood proteins cannot pass. Most patients on the artificial kidney use their machine twice a week, for about thirteen hours each time. Someone must help to "connect them up" at the start and disconnect them at the finish.

Ten years ago setting up an artificial kidney machine was a chore for a medical team of five doctors, nurses, and technicians. Keeping a patient alive on a kidney machine cost a minimum of $10,000 a year. Today a person whose kidneys have failed can run his own machine at home with the help of just one other person. The cost can be less than $1,000 a year. Of course, kidney machines aren't perfect, and they are usually expensive. So far, the cheapest unit is one developed by Dr. William G. Esmond at the University of Maryland School of Medicine. Using inexpensive plastic parts, Esmond's machine costs less than $250, and operating costs are not higher than those of other, much more expensive machines. Almost a hundred patients are now on Esmond's machines, and he recently celebrated his ten-thousandth treatment.

Lack of kidney machines, and lack of trained people to administer them, today limits the treatment to only 10 percent of those who need it. Twenty thousand persons who might have been helped die yearly because they do not have access to the equipment. Committees of laymen around the country literally have the power of life and death in their allocation of these scarce resources.

The *Kelleher Rotary Respirator* is the modern version of the "iron lung." When using this equipment, the patient lies under a removable lid, with only his head outside the chamber of the machine. A pump sucks air out of the chamber, and the reduced pressure causes his chest to expand. The reduction in pressure automatically expands the lungs—which then draw air through the patient's nose. Then the pump reverses the process and the air is expelled.

Adults usually breathe about eighteen times a minute, but the respirators can be adjusted to individual rates. The body also can be turned and tilted automatically to help drain liquid blocking the lungs—which would normally be done by coughing. For less serious cases there are respirators that allow the patient to move; some force air into the lungs through a tube inserted into the windpipe through the neck; others have a curved breastplate which works on the pressure principle of the big respirator. Their pump units are small enough to attach to wheelchairs.

The respirator unquestionably will be around for a long time. To some extent because of size, it's distinctly more difficult to make an artificial lung than to make an artificial heart.

The *heart-lung* machine, first used in the early 1950s, has changed heart surgery drastically. The arteries and veins leading into and out of the heart are clamped and plastic tubes are inserted into them. Deoxygenated blood is drawn away from the heart into the machine. There it is oxygenated while air bubbles are removed. The blood is then warmed and pumped back to the great artery arising from the left chamber of the heart (the aorta). None of the blood enters the heart chambers, and since the machine oxygenates the blood, the lungs stop working. Thus, two of man's most vital organs—heart and lungs—are temporarily replaced by a man-made organ.

The entire switch from normal to artificial living generally takes less than sixty seconds, but it requires a highly trained team of technicians, anesthesiologists, surgeons, and hematologists, working in disciplined partnership. Today, heart-lungs exist only in operating theaters; tomorrow they may be used on the wards to give weakened hearts a chance to rest and recuperate. Indeed, American scientists are already perfecting small implantable pumps that will be able to do the same job. Say you're feeling a little tired at your desk in 1990; you switch on the miniaturized heart-lung machine that's been implanted in your chest, and your entire system gets a rest for fifteen minutes while the mechanical one takes over.

Sometime in the 1970s we are probably going to produce a

successful *artificial heart*. The research budget for this is roughly $70 million each year. One might argue that this money could be used for food for a lot of undernourished children, but our problem-solving technicians argue back that the money wouldn't be spent for food, anyway.

About half a million persons yearly might be candidates for new hearts. And only ten thousand die annually from brain injury. Clearly, the future of transplant lies statistically in favor of the development of mechanical artificial hearts. Someday they may be as common as hearing aids. ("Say, Ed, can I use your desk today? I'm recharging my new Model 63 heart, and you're nearer the outlet.")

In April, 1969, an artificial heart made of fiber and plastic kept a Skokie, Illinois, man alive for sixty-five hours until a human donor was found. The patient, Haskell Karp, who died in Houston after receiving a human heart, was the first person to have an artificial heart implanted into his chest to replace his original heart. It was powered by an electrical source outside his body.

Three eminent surgeons, Adrian Kantrowitz, Michael DeBakey, and Willen Kolff, have already made sensational progress. DeBakey has lived to see his heart "stolen" by his former protégé, the flamboyant Dr. Denton Cooley. Kolff's experimental synthetic heart is the most realistic of current artificial hearts. Made of silicone, it has four chambers, four valves, and two main arteries. The walls are layered so that when the heart is connected to a machine, rhythmic spurts of air are pumped between the layers.

But the remaining research problems are vast. Materials

must be found which neither destroy blood cells nor form blood clots. A perfectly synchronized and harmonious pumping action has yet to be developed, so that a power source planted inside the body could keep the heart pumping seventy-five times per minute, thirty million times each year. Among the suggested implantable power sources are nuclear-driven miniaturized steam engines and electrohydraulic units.

To be completely satisfactory as a replacement for the human heart, a mechanical device must be made of a material which has considerable elasticity and which prevents the natural tendency of blood to clot when it touches a foreign substance. Since 1964, the National Heart and Lung Institute has spent more than $20 million on contracts to universities, hospitals, and electronic, chemical, and engineering firms in an effort to develop a workable artificial heart. It believes that a completely robot heart, once considered an impossible dream, is now "not at all far-fetched."

Dr. Frank Hastings, director of NHLI's Artificial Heart Program, said that contracts are being let in four areas: material, power mechanisms, energy source controls, and physiological problems. (For example, there are currently twenty organizations working on blood-compatible materials.) He expects a total heart device before 1980.

The use of *electrical forces* in medicine is not new. For years the electroencephalograph has been able to pick up "brain waves"—the electrical output of the brain. The readings taken on such equipment can tell psychiatrists and other qualified readers a great deal about a person's mental state—indeed, whether he even has one!

Electrocardiograms take readings of the condition of the heart, and electroshock can restart a stopped heart or stimulate some other response in a mentally ill patient.

Public interest in organ transplants has tended to obscure the at least equally bright promise of what are called heart-assist devices. Such equipment is likely to be even more important than transplant in the future treatment of heart disease. For example, the *heart pacemaker* was the first electronic device implanted to substitute for faulty nerve functions. Supreme Court Justice William O. Douglas wears one of these. The pacemaker's job is to shock the heart into regular beats. Advances in miniaturization of implantable electronic parts since the first pacemaker have been both tremendously exciting and a little frightening.

The electronic pacemakers that keep the hearts of thousands of persons with chronic cardiac disease beating have one major fault—the batteries that power them run down every eighteen to thirty months. At best, the patient must undergo periodic surgery to install a replacement; the worst could be sudden death. Recently, a French team announced that it had developed and was implanting a nuclear-powered pacemaker guaranteed for ten years. The device, designed by Dr. Paul Laurens of Broussais Hospital in Paris, has some very special new properties. Most pacemakers generate a steady impulse that keeps the heart rate at a preset level. Laurens' device is a sophisticated "demand" pacemaker. When the natural heartbeat is sufficient to pump blood, it remains inoperative. But as the heart rhythm lags, the pacemaker automatically takes over. Consequently, the pacemaker might last as long as a lifetime.

Different research by Dr. Adrian Kantrowitz, of Maimonides Hospital in Brooklyn, New York, has produced an electronic stimulator to help paraplegics who have lost normal *bladder control.* An electronic device is placed inside the abdomen in a "pocket" made just below the navel. From there, two wires lead down to the walls of the bladder. To empty the bladder, the patient holds a portable transmitter exactly over the spot where the device lies in the abdomen and presses a button. The required stimulus is then automatically applied to the bladder mechanics, and the paraplegic urinates.

Kantrowitz is also working on an electronic device to shock a particular nerve to provoke a response in the diaphragm. If this experiment succeeds, the normal breathing movements of the diaphragm could be electrically initiated, and the need for iron lungs eliminated.

*Electronic "eyes"* are also the subject of research in a number of countries. In Mexico, Dr. Armando del Campo, a psychiatrist at the National University, has developed an apparatus in which photoelectric cells on the forehead pick up light and convert it into an electrical impulse. This impulse is passed by electrodes to nerves and on to the brain. Well over a hundred patients claim to have "seen" vague images in black, gray, and white; some have even claimed to see in color. The device is not yet suitable for people who were born blind, since they have no visual memory. The messages the brain receives about the objects in front of the blind person have to be distinguishable by experience, since electronic sight is not conventional or exact. Dr. del Campo says that a tree is "seen" as a dark shadow with sparkling lights at the top and that wearers of the device can find knives or forks and distinguish between dishes on a dark tablecloth.

The next big step, after putting electrical signals into the body, has been to "take out" signals that are already there. In 1955, a research team at Guys Hospital in London worked on the possibility of using the infinitesimal amounts of electric current produced by Dr. A. H. Bottomley at West Hendon Hospital. There he developed the most refined artificial limb yet used on any amputee, the *electronic hand*.

John Cope was born with his right forearm missing from about three inches below the elbow. Nevertheless he can snip a rose from a bush easily using the Bottomley "myoelectric" hand. Bottomley chose Cope for the experiment because of his particular disability. Six hours after going into the hospital he was wearing and controlling his new hand, which is so real in appearance and so refined in control that he can pick up a dime and hand it to you without your realizing he is using an artificial hand.

Electrical impulses from the muscle activity in Cope's stump are picked up by electrodes, amplified, and fed into a tiny control unit. They are then circuited to the hand to drive it. Both amplifier and control unit are worn on a belt; both are small enough to be neither detectable nor uncomfortable.

John Cope worked for half an hour at an oscilloscope (a machine used to register electrical impulses), watching the green line flicker as he twitched his muscles. He learned to control muscles that his other arm had always used; that is, the natural set of contractions we use to transmit messages to the hand in opening and closing the first two fingers and thumb immediately. Today he is skilled in the use of the hand. When he is picking things up, Cope doesn't look at his hand but at the object he is picking up—the normal procedure. He uses his hand to gesture with, and also for smoking. Sometimes he worries: "If I have a cigarette there, it's easy to smoke right to the end without knowing it, and burn the plastic surface of the hand."

Even this problem may be solved someday, by giving artificial limbs a sense of touch. Researchers in Holland have already produced a myoelectric hand similar to Cope's, but which gives the wearer some sense of touch from the fingers! Small crystals planted in an aluminum thumb produce weak electric signals which are then amplified by tiny circuits in the hands and then transmitted to the wearer's skin and eventually to the brain.

The work on the senses and on the role of electrical impulses in muscles promises much for the future. An electronic cell which can be implanted in the muscles behind an amputated limb to trigger motions in an artificial limb is being developed. It is thought that an assembly of such cells working in the same group of muscles could reproduce the complexities of a human limb in an artificial one. In addition, paraplegics may benefit from external electrical impulses which shock useless muscles into movement. One doctor prophesied the development of a portable computer programmed with signals to send out "shock" messages to the paralyzed limbs, perhaps with miniaturized controls in the patient's pocket. In one refinement, electrodes have been implanted in the inner ear of patients when surgery failed to restore hearing, and some recipients have recognized familiar but long-unheard tunes.

New hope for paraplegics in wheelchairs, trapped by the limitations of their vehicles, has come from an unexpected quarter. The Space-General Corporation of America designed an eight-legged vehicle to stroll around the moon—appropriately enough called the Lunar Walker. A rehabilitation center in California realized its potential and is currently testing it with severely handicapped children. The walker can be operated with one hand or even a chin, and a single control stick can electrically turn the vehicle to the left or right, put it into forward or reverse. The greatest asset the children have discovered is that they can now climb stairs independently. In fact, they can even take a trip to the beach alone; since the walker has been designed to cope with the soft surfaces of the moon, it takes sand in eight-legged stride. Technologists feel that with certain modifications the lunar walker will soon be taking handicapped earthlings into a new world of freedom long before it is used by astronauts to explore their realms of outer space. In short, the control of nervous complaints by electronics is in its earliest stages, but the medical potential is overwhelming.

# The Last Word:
## Immortality?

*I wish it were possible to invent a method of embalming dead persons in such a manner that they may be recalled to life at any period . . . for having a very ardent desire to see and observe the state of America a hundred years hence.*

—Benjamin Franklin

# HOPE FOR THE FUTURE

*Freeze—Wait—Re-animate!*

—Motto of the Life Extension Society

Dr. Robert C. W. Ettinger may have the last word on rejuvenation, for Ettinger believes not merely that rejuvenation is possible, but that *immortality* itself is the only reasonable goal. A professor of physics at Highland Park College, Michigan, Ettinger believes that a panicky search for rejuvenation is irrelevant. As he sees it, all we need do today is have ourselves deep-frozen against that day—certainly inevitable—when medical science will have cured all mankind's ills. His case is convincingly set forth in his best-selling *The Prospect of Immortality*, a book that has won him devotees all over the world. He has assembled a reputable scientific advisory board whose members offer technical assistance and advice where possible, and who classify themselves as open-minded to Ettinger's claims, or at least as "unopposed." "After all," says Ettinger, "the freezer program is just another medical measure to prolong life—hardly more bizarre than an iron lung, hardly more unnatural than penicillin, hardly more radical than kidney transplant."

A bewildering array of special-interest groups have capitalized on Ettinger's proposals, the most notable being the Cryonics Society and the Life Extension Society. Branches of these organizations now exist all over the United States—indeed, all over the world. They have been working hard to get support from the general public and professional people for a wide-ranging "freezer program" that would throw every-

**173**

body into sub-zero at the opportune time until cures can be found for their illnesses, including aging itself.

Many believers have made provision in their wills to have themselves and their families quick-frozen and stored for future rescue. Since they are dying anyway, clearly they have nothing to lose. Some new firms have designed insulated caskets for this specific purpose. Entrepreneurs are peddling "cryocapsules" for $15,000 each, plus $1,550 yearly storage. Contractees are hermetically sealed in an eleven-foot cushion suspended over 150 gallons of liquid nitrogen, the fumes of which continually circulate about the "corpse."

The first known cryonic freeze took place on January 12, 1966, when the body of psychologist Dr. James Bedford was frozen by a team of doctors in Glendale, California, and freighted in a sealed cryocapsule to Phoenix, Arizona, where he is currently being stored at 320° F. below zero, a temperature maintained by liquid nitrogen. Since Bedford, thousands have registered their desire to be buried in this fashion with the Cryonics Society of America. Members carry cards and Medic Alert wristbands with emergency freezing instructions explaining the procedure necessary in case of death. Some chapters of the Cryonics Society have even fitted out mobile rescue units equipped for quick-freezing.

As of July 21, 1970, thirteen persons had been so frozen, and members of the "establishment" are taking a fresh interest in cryonics.

The largest permanent storage facility to date has been built by Cryonic Interment, Inc., in a cemetery near Los Angeles. Minnesota Valley Engineering Company, a very reputable firm, has undertaken a new program for the manufacture of a new type of cryocapsule or "forever flask" that will keep patients permanently stored in liquid nitrogen. Certain persons have even been "installed" with the blessings of their family priest and bishop. When Mrs. Carmen DeBlasio was so stored, her unit was consecrated by Father Saverio Mattei, with the approval of the bishop. And a bill has been drafted in the Wisconsin legislature for the recognition and separate control of cryogenic interment, which the attorney general of that state has already ruled legal.

All of the separate nonprofit cryonics societies, most of them regional, have now banded together under the banner of the Cryonics Society of America. Annual prizes are awarded for the most outstanding research in cryobiology. Several years ago a prize went to Professor Isamu Suda and his colleagues at Kobe University for long-term freezing of cat brains which survived.

Interest in cryonics is also increasing rapidly overseas. There are now two cryonics societies in France, and one each in Germany, Spain, Brazil, and Colombia. A brief glance at the roster of any cryonics meeting shows a considerable list of qualified scientists from every field—geologists, anatomists, physicians, anthropologists, chemists, biologists, engineers, management counselors, educators, physicists, lawyers, psychologists. They are from Litton Industries, the California Institute of Technology, Tulane, Harvard, University of California, Raytheon Corporation, the Department of Health, Education, and Welfare, Northwestern University, and other centers of progress.

Can we survive freezing and thawing? Even Ettinger admits that we can't—not yet: "With present methods, not completely. But with future methods of thawing and repair, it may be possible to rescue even those frozen by crude methods. With the best of [current] methods, there may be relatively little freezing damage." Can revival after freezing be guaranteed? Ettinger says: "No. But we can guarantee that, if you are not frozen, you will not be revived. We can also guarantee that, if you are frozen and not revived, you will be no worse off."

If man should ever become immortal, society will face some tremendous new problems because our entire philosophy has been geared to a brief existence. Our entire life orientation will have to change. Political leaders clinging to power may never die. Wealth and power may gradually gravitate to the old. There may be no inheritances, no selling of businesses "due to retirement." Periodic and bloody revolutions by the younger population may have to occur if they are to gain power.

It may be that immortality will mean unlimited boredom. If men and women can have children at any time, they may elect to put off having them and children may become a distinct rarity. The sheer endlessness of life may cause the ambitious to lose their ambition. There may be no great rush for success or status if they may be had at any time in an endless future—they may not provide enough solid gratification to be worth the effort. Possibly the immortals may do something totally unexpected—curse this infinite life and long for death, even commit suicide.

If the U.S. Congress were to retain the seniority system, what would this mean in an age when congressmen live for thousands of years? Would vigorous ancients keep the reins of politics, business, and family finances, frustrating the young? Would conflict between the generations supersede hostility between classes and races? Would insurance and pension plans continue payments forever? Would aging control become as vital as birth control? The changes wrought in our society with the advent of immortality would exceed those brought about by splitting the atom or man's voyages to the moon.

# Here and Now

*What is life? It is a flash of a firefly in the night. It is a breath of a buffalo in the winter time. It is as the little shadow that runs across the grass and loses itself in the sunset.*

—Isapwo Muksika, Crowfoot chief, 1890

Does death require a new definition? Is legalized euthanasia an answer? Or is there another hope for the future? Is rejuvenation possible? Even more to the point: Is immortality a reasonable subject for scientific pursuit?

Today the outlook for the aged who are terminally ill is anything but promising, and we lack the brilliance to propound world-saving theories, any of which would be faced with the immense inertia that is the real world. What can one man do, or even several? The system of dying was constructed by our culture, which shows no indication of seeking to overhaul itself.

NTBR decisions are commonplace among doctors and nurses in *every* hospital. They are taken for granted. So much so, in fact, that a researcher feels naive and silly poking around for information. Only the traditional lack of communication between medicine and the public it ostensibly serves obscures this obviousness.

The final point of this book is simply that if one does not arrange one's own date with death, the arrangements will be made by strangers and others who fundamentally don't give a damn.

## CROSSING THE BAR

SUNSET and evening star,
    And one clear call for me!
And may there be no moaning of the bar,
    When I put out to sea,

## THE GODS OF LIFE

But such a tide as moving seems asleep,
    Too full for sound and foam,
When that which drew from out the boundless deep
    Turns again home.

Twilight and evening bell,
    And after that the dark!
And may there be no sadness of farewell,
    When I embark;

For tho' from out our bourne of Time and Place
    The flood may bear me far,
I hope to see my Pilot face to face
    When I have crossed the bar.

*Alfred, Lord Tennyson*

N.E.

| ECHEANCE | DATE DUE |
|---|---|
| FEB 1 4 1978 β | FEB 4 1988 β |
| 4/7/78 β | DEC 0 8 1991 β |
| | MAR - 2 1992 β |
| DEC 1 4 1978 β | MAR 2 5 1992 |
| DEC 2 0 1978 β | Apr 15 β |
| MAY 1 6 1979 β | MAY 1 4 1992 β |
| DEC 1 8 1979 | FEB - 9 1993 βυ |
| MAR - 2 1982 β | |
| APR 2 2 1983 β | NOV 0 8 1993 MR |
| JUN _ 7 1983 | MAR 1 5 1994 AB |
| JUN 1 3 1983 | NOV 0 9 1994 |
| | MAR 3 0 1995 G |
| DEFERRED - A PLUS TARD | |
| DEC 0 5 1986 | |

Université de Sudbury
University of Sudbury